Sexual Behaviour and AIDS in the Developing World

Social Aspects of AIDS

Series Editor: Peter Aggleton
Institute of Education, University of London

Sexual Behaviour and AIDS in the Developing World

Edited by

John Cleland and Benoît Ferry

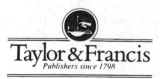

Taylor & Francis
Publishers since 1798

WORLD HEALTH ORGANIZATION

UK   Taylor & Francis Ltd, 4 John St., London WC1N 2ET
USA   Taylor & Francis Inc., 1900 Frost Road, Suite 101, Bristol, PA 19007

First published 1995

A Catalogue Record for this book is available from the British Library

ISBN 0 7484 0343 4
ISBN 0 7484 0344 2 pbk

Library of Congress Cataloging-in-Publication Data are available on request

Series cover design by Barking Dog Art, additional artwork by Hybert • Design & Type.

Typeset in 10/12pt Baskerville
by Graphicraft Typesetters Ltd., Hong Kong

Printed in Great Britain by Burgess Science Press, Basingstoke, on paper which has a specified pH value on final paper manufacture of not less than 7.5 and is therefore 'acid free'.

Contents

Contents

List of Tables

List of Figures

Foreword

Social and behavioural research on AIDS is of critical importance to the design of effective interventions for prevention, as well as to their evaluation. Such has been recognized by international and national agencies, many of which have devoted considerable resources to the support of social and behavioural research in developing and developed countries. From the earliest days of the epidemic, the World Health Organization's Global Programme on AIDS has invested heavily in this field so as to enable the development of more effective programmes.

Initially, this enquiry took the form of studies of HIV and AIDS-related knowledge, attitudes and behaviours. These studies were intended to provide much needed information about risk behaviours and their determinants, as well as baseline data against which to judge the effectiveness of behavioural interventions. More recently, the focus has broadened to examine the contexts within which risk-related behaviour occurs, as well as the social consequences of the epidemic for individuals and for affected communities.

Given that unprotected sex accounts for by far the greatest number of infections worldwide, the decision to focus on patterns of sexual behaviour was appropriate. When the Global Programme on AIDS came into being, little was known about patterns of sexual behaviour in developing countries in Africa, Asia and Central and South America. When planning HIV prevention and care, policy makers and programme planners therefore had to rely either on stereotype and supposition, or on findings from studies conducted for other purposes. It was within this context that the World Health Organization decided to support the series of studies of HIV and AIDS-related knowledge, attitudes and reported behaviours in developing countries which are described in this book.

While the primary purpose of these studies was to inform national efforts in the fields of prevention and care, their use of similar methods of data collection and analysis enabled across-site comparisons to be made. This is the first global report of its kind to contain inter-country comparisons of HIV and AIDS-related knowledge, attitudes and behaviour in the developing world.

A multi-site study such as this facilitates critical reflection on the strengths and weaknesses of this style of social enquiry, particularly as it relates to work in the field of HIV and AIDS. The authors and editors do not shy away from this task, either methodologically or substantively. Instead, they offer a balanced assessment of what population surveys can offer, recognizing that in the absence of additional contextual information generated through parallel kinds of enquiry, the interpretation of findings will tell only part of the story. And here lies the challenge for the social sciences in the years ahead – to design and conduct local investigations which hold the potential to lead to better interventions in both prevention and care.

Michael Merson
Executive Director
World Health Organization
Global Programme on AIDS

Preface

This volume contains findings from sexual behaviour and partner relations surveys conducted in the late 1980s and early 1990s in countries in Sub-Saharan Africa, Asia, and Central and South America. A total of 16 surveys are reported on here. This unique data collection effort was begun in 1988 by the Social and Behavioural Research Unit of the World Health Organization's Global Programme on AIDS (GPA). The final data sets were assembled and analyzed by the Social and Behavioural Studies and Support Unit of the World Health Organization's Global Programme on AIDS between 1991–1994. The GPA Steering Committee on Social and Behavioural Research supports with considerable enthusiasm the publication of key findings from this programme of work. Some of the reasons for that support are:

- Prevention of HIV through behavioural change is now, and will be for the foreseeable future, the only way to prevent its spread. Even the vaccines that are likely to be developed will probably not be 100 per cent effective, requiring continued behaviour change to prevent the further spread of HIV.
- At the time the work was begun, no national surveys on sexual behaviour had been undertaken in developing countries, and surveys on AIDS-related knowledge and attitudes were sparse. It was essential therefore to collect data on sexual behaviour, partner relations and condom use to pursue this new domain for both basic science and prevention efforts.
- These multi-site studies provide the first comprehensive database on sexual behaviour in the developing world. Future studies will need to monitor sexual behaviour in various populations and measure risk behaviour changes so as to determine changing needs.
- The mapping of risk behaviour by population groups is essential for the effective targeting of prevention efforts. Further refinement of programmes will require an evolving understanding of where the epidemic is going. Background information, such as that presented here, is essential for the development of appropriate interventions and proper policies, and these need to evolve as the epidemic evolves.
- When the AIDS epidemic began, only a few sociologists, anthropologists and psychologists were involved in HIV and AIDS-related research. The studies reported here played an important role in the

development of these fields at the international level. It was essential to involve more social and behavioural scientists, given that behaviour change was the only way to prevent the spread of the epidemic. In the developing world, this initiative from the World Health Organization's Global Programme on AIDS stimulated key human resources to become more involved in AIDS research and interventions.

The surveys themselves presented an enormous challenge. It was challenging to determine the best methods for studying and measuring difficult issues such as sexual behaviour. The definition of basic concepts and their operationalization was no easy task given the lack of literature on how best to reliably and validly assess intimate behaviours. The World Health Organization's Global Programme on AIDS deliberately wanted to stimulate research that provided cross-national comparisons and meet the challenge of developing samples and sampling strategies that would allow generalization to broader populations. The completion of such projects is never easy. Only concerted and determined effort allowed the databases to be assembled, documented, and analyzed.

The findings documented here have important implications for prevention. The data provide us with a picture of variations in sexual behaviour across gender, age groups and population groups. They provide insight into factors that are, and are not, related to sexual behaviour. They also begin to tell us where to focus prevention efforts. Repeated cross-sectional surveys could yield an even a better picture of how populations are changing their behaviour and where future efforts might be best focused.

However, the work presented here is only a beginning. It was difficult to initiate due to scientific, logistical and policy problems. Such work had never been done before, and mounting cross-national surveys is difficult even with the vast experience in this working group. Studies of sexual behaviour may be uncomfortable for individuals, groups and nations, and survey studies provide only a glimpse of the behaviours studied. Clearly this work needs to be complemented with studies that use other designs, questions and approaches to provide a more complete picture of sexual risk behaviour and suggest even more effective avenues for intervention. Social and behavioural enquiry such as this, as well as a wide variety of other kinds of studies needs to be continued and supported so as to ensure that HIV and other sexually-related epidemics can be better understood and countered more effectively. The GPA Steering Committee on Social and Behavioural Research (1991–1994) is proud to have supported this work. We hope that it stimulates scientists from many disciplines to undertake sexual behaviour research, and we hope that it contributes to saving more people from the scourge of HIV.

The following are the members of the Steering Committee on Social and Behavioural Research (1991–1994) World Health Organization, Global Programme on AIDS:

Thomas J. Coates (Chair), University of California, San Francisco;

Mario P. Bronfman, El Colegio de México, Mexico D.F.;

Monica Dasgupta, National Council of Applied Economic Research, New Delhi;

Alan King, Queen's University, Ontario;

Marvelous Mhloyi, University of Zimbabwe, Harare;

Jean-Paul Moatti, Institut National de la Santé et de la Recherche Médicale, Marseille;

Arletty Pinel, São Paulo;

Werasit Sittitrai, Thai Red Cross Society, Bangkok;

Rob A. Tielman, University of Utrecht, Utrecht.

Chapter 1

History and Background

Manuel Carballo

Introduction

When the Special Programme on AIDS of the World Health Organization (WHO), later to become the Global Programme on AIDS (GPA), formally came into being in January 1987, three main areas of activity were proposed: the mobilization of interest and resources; the provision of collaborative support to national action; and the promotion of global research and interventions. They reflected what were seen as the main international needs at the time. Later, as the level of activity within these areas grew, the global research component was further broken down and units focusing on social and behavioural research, biomedical research, epidemiology and surveillance, and health promotion were set up. Until this point, much of the research that had been done on the subject of AIDS had been essentially in the biomedical domain. Most of it, moreover, continued to be undertaken in, or managed from, developed countries where resources were available and where the greatest interest in HIV and AIDS had emerged. The amount of social and behavioural research going on or planned still lagged well behind that in the biomedical sciences. Despite the fact that funds were available from many national sources, the subject of AIDS had not aroused the level of interest required for social and behavioural scientists to mount many major national, and certainly not international, initiatives.

Six years into the pandemic, and at a time when the level of political interest by countries was increasing, there thus continued to be a dearth of systematically gathered information on the psychosocial factors affecting HIV transmission and what implications these might have for society and public health in general. Given the international nature of AIDS and the fact that HIV infection was increasing, the lack of any cross-cultural comparative data was especially significant.

The dearth of information available on the social and behavioural aspects of HIV transmission was all the more marked in the case of developing countries where the prevalence of HIV infection was by then becoming more widely acknowledged. The field of health promotion was especially wanting in the type and quality of information needed to develop models of the factors affecting transmission and prevention strategies.

Little was known about how AIDS was affecting public thinking, about the ways in which people perceived the problem, or indeed what they knew about the transmission of HIV/AIDS. Even less was known in such key areas as sexual behaviour and injecting drug use. For example, there had still not been any major attempt to generate cross-cultural information on patterns of either heterosexual, homosexual, or bisexual behaviour, or to identify population-based factors that might help explain past, or project future trends in the epidemiology of HIV. It became evident that, even with respect to other more familiar sexually transmitted diseases, there had been little systematic behavioural and social science on which research could be built.

By the end of 1987, the planning requirements of National AIDS Committees and others were increasingly pointing to a need for social and behavioural information that could be used in the formulation of local AIDS policies and programmes as well as to monitor trends and evaluate interventions.

Development of Activities

Two main requirements were identified when the Social and Behavioural Research Unit (SBR) was established. The first was to respond to the need for country-specific data that might help identify psychosocial factors influencing HIV transmission; the second was to help generate a body of systematic cross-cultural information that might help explain patterns of HIV/AIDS, that would provide a foundation on which national and international monitoring might be built, and that would also constitute a behavioural base to assist in projecting future trends in the disease.

In order to help WHO/GPA define a work agenda in this area, and to ensure that it reflected the needs of a broad spectrum of disciplines, a meeting of researchers, clinicians and community health and social workers was organized at the end of 1987. The meeting concluded that four main lines of research and development were called for, with the following purposes:

- to provide explanatory models of the pandemic and to identify and describe public perceptions and knowledge about the disease;
- to define and measure high-risk behaviours associated with HIV transmission;
- to describe the types of coping responses emerging among individuals and communities;
- to identify ways in which social support and counselling could be provided in different socio-economic settings.

Within each of the above areas, the first task became one of assessing what had already been done and what research was underway in different parts of the world. Accordingly, research institutes and professional associations were contacted and literature searches undertaken. At the same time, an attempt was made to identify the results of any social and behavioural research and how they were being applied to the design and implementation of national HIV/AIDS prevention interventions.

Contact was also made with National AIDS Programmes and Committees. They were encouraged to include social and behavioural researchers as part of their membership and to become involved in setting national priorities for social and behavioural research. Local research-information meetings were organized in a large number of countries, especially in those without a strong tradition in social and behavioural research. To the extent possible, the creation of national multidisciplinary groups was promoted so that researchers and planners could exchange views and ideas about collaboration.

Priority was also given to mobilizing more interest in this general area and to encouraging international collaboration between researchers. International meetings of psychologists, sociologists, anthropologists, epidemiologists and social workers were targeted and provided with information on the unit's research agenda. Meanwhile staff of the National Programme Support Unit of GPA were also encouraged to incorporate the theme of social and behavioural research in their discussions with countries on short and medium-term AIDS plans.

In parallel, a series of technical working groups were established to help develop each of the research and development areas that had been proposed. Specifically, activities were started on the subject of knowledge, attitudes, beliefs and practices (KABP), related to AIDS; general public sexual behaviour; homosexual behaviour; bisexual behaviour; injecting drug behaviour; coping responses; and counselling. This report details the development and findings of the General Public KABP and Sexual Behaviour surveys.

Knowledge, Attitudes, Beliefs and Practices

Surveys of the knowledge (K) people have about selected health issues, their attitudes (A) to them and their subsequent practices (P), were not new. For example, in the area of family planning, where attitudinal and behavioural change is a major concern, KAP surveys began to be used widely in the early 1970s. However, their success in predicting contraceptive adoption varied considerably and attempts to use standardized methods in different countries often met with difficulties of acceptance, comprehension and meaning. As a result, KAP surveys began to be criticized, and during the course of the 1970s the frequency of their use diminished.

Given that attitudinal and behavioural change would necessarily have to be an integral part of AIDS prevention, however, the development of research on knowledge, attitudes and practices (KAP) was again taken up as a basis for designing and evaluating interventions. In preparing the WHO/GPA survey instruments, previous experiences with KAP research were critically reviewed and a strategy prepared to help overcome some of the problems that had been encountered in KAP surveys on other subjects. Because of the need to provide a broad account of how people respond to AIDS and information about it, a decision was taken to add a *beliefs* component to the traditional KAP approach.

One of the main concerns in the KABP surveys was to be able to define concepts and measures that could be usefully applied in as many cultural contexts as possible. Much previous work of this type had been focused on single cultures and there was little experience to build on with respect to cross-culturally comparative research. For this reason, care was taken to bring together social psychologists, anthropologists and sociologists with research experience in as broad a range of cultures as possible.

Sexual Behaviour

Within the area of sexual behaviour, the design of population-based surveys was even more complex. The provision of national baseline and, at the same time, cross-culturally comparative information, presented a number of conceptual, methodological and logistical challenges. The Kinsey survey of sexual behaviour in the United States (Kinsey, 1948; 1953) was by then over 20 years old and relatively outdated because of subsequent changes in sexual behaviour. Moreover, parts of it had been criticized for reasons of in-built biases and it was generally held to offer little that could be easily extrapolated to the current AIDS pandemic. The only other major survey that might have been relevant was the World Fertility Survey[1] which had been conducted some ten years earlier. This had looked at fertility determinants and contraceptive behaviour, but had not taken up questions of human sexuality (except on post-partum abstinence, onset of sexual activity and frequency of sexual intercourse) and thus has thrown little light on the behavioural dimensions relevant to AIDS. Similarly, the successor to the World Fertility Survey, the Demographic and Health Survey[2], did not address the topic of HIV transmission before the inclusion of a few questions relevant to HIV/AIDS in its recent surveys.

The apparent lack of interest in the study of sexual behaviour reflected the many methodological and cultural constraints involved. There were important concerns about how to reach and involve people in providing reliable information on private and sensitive topics. At the same time there were also concerns about the political acceptability of research in this area, especially in countries with little tradition of sample surveys and, in particular, with little tradition of open discussion of sexuality. Even as it was becoming increasingly clear that information about human sexuality was basic to understanding HIV transmission, there were expressions about how difficult, even impossible, it would be to undertake cross-cultural work on the subject.

The working group that was set up to help develop the sexual behaviour instruments thus needed to bring together a variety of skills and experiences.

Not only were sociologists, demographers, psychologists and anthropologists involved but there were consultations with political scientists and clinicians too. Because of the anticipated problems of obtaining detailed information on sexuality by means of large surveys, the group was also asked to address the role of other, smaller scale but more intensive methods of gathering information.

The feasibility of doing cross-cultural sexual behaviour surveys was taken up first through a series of exploratory meetings in all the WHO regions. Working with the AIDS focal points in regional offices, a broad multi-disciplinary mix of researchers, health and social service staff, local leaders and AIDS Committee personnel were invited to review and discuss the topics being proposed for study.

Methodology

A number of key methodological questions had to be resolved early in the development of the surveys. It was agreed, for example, that the surveys could not possibly go into the type of detail required on all aspects and that complementary qualitative studies would be indispensable. The latter would provide more in-depth insights into the apparent differences in individual behaviours and help explain any group differences that might emerge. A number of additional working group meetings were therefore organized to address the need for qualitative research guidelines in all the areas identified for study; anthropologists with experience working in different parts of the world were invited to help.

Again, because the topics of human sexuality and perception were considered to be highly private and open to methodological problems, the question of reliability and validity was introduced early in the agendas of the working groups. It was decided to ensure that these concerns were addressed in the design of the main surveys themselves, and, in addition, to set up a series of independent field tests of data quality.

As a result of these discussions, a general consensus emerged that, in the first stages of the proposed work, the situation in industrialized countries might lend itself to more detailed and longer studies than in some of the more traditional societies. As a result, it was decided that, while the generic themes of both the sexual behaviour and the KABP surveys should be pursued everywhere, more expanded versions of the basic questionnaires could be proposed in industrialized societies.

In some countries, where a decision was taken early on to conduct both the KABP and sexual behaviour surveys, which for political as well as technical purposes became named the Partner Relations Surveys (PRS), it was also agreed that the interview schedules could be merged without too much loss of detail in either area. Consultations with local research staff were held wherever this was proposed and a new generic model schedule and methodology were prepared to facilitate the work at country level.

At different stages in the development of the methodologies and interview schedules for each of the KABP, the PR and the combined surveys, steps were taken to pre-test the instruments and 13 countries participated in these phases. All the researchers involved in pre-testing the questionnaires and study methods met together before and after pre-tests to discuss the ways in which they had been conducted and the results acquired.

In the case of the PR, the pre-test experience in all the participating countries pointed to a greater than anticipated willingness on the part of respondents to discuss and provide information on personal behaviour. Indeed one of the ancillary findings was the desire on the part of many people to have more information about human sexuality and to have opportunities to discuss their own sexuality with experts. Even in parts of the Eastern Mediterranean and Africa, where initially it had been suggested that research of this kind could not be carried out, the response was overwhelmingly favourable.

The pre-testing exercise also permitted WHO/GPA to identify the main logistical, equipment and financial needs of the different research groups and centres. Support needs for sampling design, data handling and analysis also began to be enumerated, and plans were formulated to respond to them. For example, while in some of the countries census tract information was available, others had no well established base of this kind to build on. In some, data handling facilities were readily available, while in others it became clear that it would be essential to build up a data analysis capability.

Regional Organization

WHO regional offices were encouraged to participate with WHO/GPA headquarters in Geneva in all phases of project development. As well as the initial exploratory meetings in the regions, a series of more detailed research methodology meetings was organized with regional and national AIDS programme staff. These made it possible to identify experienced researchers and research institutions in the different regions, and permitted WHO/GPA to involve national scientists who had not yet had much opportunity to work on the subject of AIDS. These meetings also allowed WHO/GPA to further explain and spread information about the goals and objectives of the research agenda within countries and among senior policymakers. In some cases the meetings also provided insights into local unpublished research relevant to sexually transmitted diseases and permitted an evaluation of its potential contribution to the new research being proposed.

Moreover, these regional meetings aimed to ensure that the research agenda received the degree of legitimation and commitment needed to ensure successful implementation. In many instances, regional office staff were also able to suggest additional ways in which potential problems of a cultural or political nature might be avoided or lessened, including discussions with key political or cultural gate-keepers. This was especially important in countries where the AIDS pandemic had not necessarily been acknowledged, and where the prevalence of infection was either unknown or still low.

By March 1990, at least two and, in some cases, three research meetings had been organized in collaboration with WHO regional offices, and over 200 potential researchers had been involved. Interest in the proposed research quickly mounted in developed countries, and in the European region a number of meetings were co-sponsored with the EEC which gave rise to additional networking of technical support for national and cross-national projects.

Technical and Financial Support

As a result of these extensive preparatory activities, the study designs, protocols and questionnaires that were developed were readily adopted by countries. In France, the United Kingdom, Spain, Belgium, Netherlands and Greece, additional funds were provided by national research councils to support the work. In the United States the Partner Relations and the KABP surveys prompted new interest in this area, and a number of institutes such as the National Institute of Child Health and Development and the National Institute of Statistics adapted parts of the research instruments for incorporation in national surveys.

Elsewhere, WHO/GPA assumed responsibility for total or seed funding. In a number of countries, the research activities proposed by the countries were included within the short or medium-term plans. This was especially the case with the KABP surveys whose database was considered to be of immediate relevance to monitoring trends in the perception of AIDS, and to evaluating national interventions for AIDS prevention.

Direct funding to countries also came from bilateral sources, and in a number of African and Latin American countries, donor agencies contributed to some of the national research in terms of human as well as financial resources.

For a variety of reasons it was felt that the research should be carried out by national teams, as far as possible. This would be a way of strengthening the institutional basis for AIDS research and prevention within countries. It was also felt that on sensitive issues such as AIDS and sexual behaviour, the local knowledge of national researchers should be utilized, and that they should be the ones to determine when and how (within previously set out and agreed upon parameters) to adapt the generic protocols. Because of the need to establish databases from which long-term monitoring and evaluation could be carried out, and to undertake repeat surveys over time wherever possible, it was again thought that local researchers should be involved as early as possible in the design and implementation phases of the national projects, since, ideally, they would be the ones to implement later activities.

One of the problems created by this decision to emphasize the involvement of national researchers was that, in countries without a strong tradition of social and behavioural research, there were few researchers available. Those capable scientists with relevant experience were invariably in high demand, and few had considered this new area of AIDS research. In some instances it became necessary to visit countries to encourage ministries of health and universities to free key researchers from other responsibilities and provide them with more staff support.

Briefing and training national research staff on the techniques being proposed for the KABP and sexual behaviour surveys became an important part of this early phase of the work, and training meetings with researchers were set up in all the WHO regions during 1988 and 1989. Many of these meetings provided additional opportunities for refinement of the protocols and questionnaires. However, the meetings were primarily designed to address issues of sampling and fieldworker training.

Training on interviewing techniques was particularly necessary in countries where health surveys had not been previously undertaken and where the teams had little experience with household surveys. From an institution and research strengthening perspective it was also important to ensure that data handling and primary analysis and reporting be done at the local level. To standardize as much of this as possible, and again support local institutions, the training activities dedicated a proportion of their time to data entry and tabulation exercises. In most of the countries where personal computers were not normally available to the research teams, everything was done to provide them, be it through direct grants from WHO/GPA or through National Programme Support.

Through National AIDS Programmes and Committees, professional meetings, and direct communication with known or recommended research teams, invitations to submit proposals were put out in most developing countries and selected industrialized ones. The guidelines for proposals were structured to ensure that the priorities and minimum requirements set out by the GPA/SBR Unit could be addressed, while at the same time meeting more specific national or local needs.

Reviews of proposals were undertaken within WHO and by teams of reviewers selected for their experience with national survey development. Where proposals did not meet the requirements set out by GPA/SBR Unit, steps were taken to provide the research teams submitting the proposals with technical support so that the projects could be re-formulated and re-submitted. Consultants visiting countries with this purpose, however, were also asked to review the proposals with the National AIDS Programmes and Committees so as to ensure their active participation in the planning of research and their commitment to the project and the use of findings.

In all the regions, an assurance was given to the research teams that technical support would be made available at any point during the projects, and a number of consultant visits were made at the request of some of the national teams to assist with sampling difficulties and with data handling. In this regard a series of tabulation plans was constructed and instructions were provided with respect to data entry using as standardized an approach as possible.

Regular technical monitoring of all the projects was instituted, and visits were made to centres by consultants to ensure that the protocols and other proposed standard procedures were being followed. Visits by consultants and WHO/GPA staff permitted the researchers opportunities to discuss methodological concerns and financial problems. In a number of sites, additional funding needs emerged, and original time plans proved to be difficult to maintain in a few countries. Where this was the case it often reflected additional demands being placed on the researchers by the National AIDS Programmes and Committees and ministries, and it became clear that the KABP and the Partner Relations research projects were quickly attracting the attention of national and international groups. Not only did this research thereby become legitimized, but it accelerated interest in other related research areas, and by other national and international groups.

As indicated above, a key principle was to encourage and facilitate the handling of data and primary analysis at the country level by the national research teams themselves. To assist in this, a series of guidelines and instructions were prepared and provided to all researchers. In addition, it was decided to link selected statistical support groups with national researchers and maintain their operational relationship for as long as necessary. This continuity of support was intended to enhance technical co-operation and maintain sound technical links between researchers and support staff. Using the proposed standardized data entry procedures and data tabulation systems, it also became possible to facilitate the movement of data for secondary analysis to WHO/GPA headquarters in Geneva or other selected centres.

Results of many of these studies have already been extensively published in the international scientific literature. This volume will focus on an in-depth comparative analysis of 16 surveys undertaken in developing countries and coordinated by WHO/GPA.

Notes

1 The World Fertility Survey (WFS) conducted 42 national surveys from 1972 to 1984. It was jointly funded by UNFPA and USAID.
2 The Demographic and Health Surveys (DHS) programme is undertaken by Macro International Inc. and funded by USAID since the mid-1980s. It is designed to collect data on fertility, family planning, and maternal and child health in the developing world. By 1994, about 50 surveys had been undertaken.

Chapter 2

Characteristics of Surveys and Data Quality

Benoît Ferry with Jean-Claude Deheneffe,
Masuma Mamdani and Roger Ingham

Objectives and Content of Survey Protocols

As described in the previous chapter, WHO/GPA developed research protocols for KABP and sexual behaviour (Partner Relations) surveys. These research packages were designed to assist researchers in conducting population surveys at national or sub-national level. They consisted of a general introduction, guidelines on study design, including sampling, a model questionnaire, an interviewers' manual, a data management manual and guidelines on tabulation of data. This standardized approach was necessary to generate information that would be comparable between countries.

Research Packages on KABP and on Partner Relations (PR) were developed by WHO/GPA for the African region (Phase I) and for the rest of the world (Phase II). They were produced in English, French and Spanish. A package combining PR/KABP approaches was also prepared in English (WHO/GPA, 1990 a-e). The ultimate objectives of the surveys were to generate the data required for a better understanding of the information and education needs of various segments of the general population, and to provide the necessary baseline data for the evaluation of health promotion activities and other initiatives carried out as part of National AIDS Programmes.

The primary goal of the KABP surveys was to provide descriptive information about knowledge, attitudes, beliefs and certain behaviours in general adult populations with regard to HIV/AIDS and to facilitate, improve and evaluate HIV/AIDS prevention control activities. Specifically the KABP surveys aimed to:

- ascertain knowledge about HIV infection and AIDS;
- assess attitudes to and beliefs about HIV infection and AIDS;
- assess attitudes towards people with AIDS;
- assess awareness of the relationship between certain behaviours and HIV infection;

- identify the main sources of AIDS information and education;
- collect basic data on the relative prevalence of selected behaviours associated with risks of HIV infection;
- determine the nature and extent of behavioural changes that may have already taken place or were planned in response to AIDS;
- determine use of condoms as a means of risk reduction;
- analyze the relationship between the cognitive, attitudinal and behavioural factors described above and socio-demographic and other characteristics.

The goals of the PR surveys were broadly similar to those of KABP surveys, but with a greater emphasis on the measurement of sexual behaviours that carry a potential risk of HIV infection. It should be noted that neither KABP nor PR investigations were designed to evaluate any specific theory. Rather they were intended to meet a wide range of pragmatic information needs. This orientation reflects the strengths and limitations of large scale surveys compared to other types of research. It is almost impossible to meet the data requirements of any theory within the restrictions of a single-round survey, even if consensus could be reached on an appropriate theoretical framework.

The core questionnaire for both KABP and PR surveys consisted of two parts: a household or dwelling identification part, and a much longer part to be administered to individual men and women aged 15 to 49 years. The main purpose of the household form was to identify individuals eligible for the detailed personal interview. Generally it was not processed. The longer individual part was made up of core sections. These were expected to take about 45 minutes to complete. The topics covered in the questionnaire are discussed below.

Background Characteristics for KABP and PR Surveys

Both types of questionnaire started with standard and relatively innocuous questions about the background of respondents. One purpose of this ordering was to establish rapport before more sensitive issues were broached. Details about the respondent include such characteristics as education, employment, mobility and religion. A number of variables were included in order to permit an analysis of knowledge, attitudes, beliefs and practices within the broader social context in which they occurred. Other variables were measured because of their possible influence on, and association with behaviour: these included such items as religion and religiosity, urban-rural status, and mobility and temporary migration. Similarly, exposure to mass media was included because of its potential role in determining knowledge, attitudes and beliefs. In many countries, a key component of HIV/AIDS control and prevention strategies are mass media initiatives. Three specific items of information were included: frequency of newspaper readership, radio listening and television viewing. Following this common introductory content, the main sections of KABP and PR questionnaires diverged. The content of the KABP instrument will be described first.

KABP Instrument

Awareness of AIDS

Because AIDS is a relatively new problem, not all respondents have the awareness needed for attitude formation. This section was therefore designed to establish awareness of AIDS so that those who are unaware could be excluded from further questions on detailed knowledge and understanding, and on attitudes.

Although the local investigators were encouraged to adapt the questionnaires to allow for local variation in the terminology used (for example, using *slim disease* instead of AIDS), the use of terms from developed countries in quite different settings creates unavoidable problems. Thus, reporting that one is 'aware of AIDS' in a European or North American country probably reflects having heard of the term (through the media and/or other source) and having some set of associations or social representations for which it stands. These can then be further examined through closer questioning of those who report being aware of the 'condition'. On the other hand, in cultures and sub-cultures where access to mass media is not widespread, or where lay understandings of illness, infection, and other medical terms are not as objectified as they are in Western countries, this question might have different meanings and associations. The existence of different perspectives is a difficult issue to overcome in questionnaire-based survey work in different cultures, especially where attempts are made to use standardized instruments.

Knowledge of AIDS

As a central theme of the investigation, this topic was covered by a relatively large number of questions dealing with respondents' knowledge of various aspects of HIV infection and AIDS: causation, routes of transmission, the infectious status of affected individuals, fatality, groups at risk, cure, and so on. While most of the knowledge items were designed to identify specific areas of misinformation that needed to be considered in formulating a health promotion campaign, the responses to these items could be analysed together to form a single *Knowledge-of-AIDS-scale* for use in multivariate analyses and comparisons of social groups and subgroups.

Attitudes to AIDS

A distinction was made between attitudes to AIDS as a disease or health problem, and attitudes towards people with HIV infection or AIDS, including their care, treatment and management.

Beliefs about AIDS

Two distinct beliefs regarding AIDS and other health problems were expected to be of major significance in determining behavioural response: the perceived seriousness of AIDS and perceived personal vulnerability to AIDS. If individuals did not regard AIDS as an important problem and/or did not think that they were personally at risk of HIV infection, the chances of changing behaviour in response to AIDS information might be low. These two beliefs were assessed through a number of questions.

Behavioural Responses to AIDS

Two different aspects of this topic were covered in the core sections of the questionnaire: awareness that certain behaviours might expose individuals to risk of HIV infection, and willingness to avoid risk by changing behaviour. A series of questions covered these two aspects of behavioural response to AIDS.

Contraceptive Knowledge and Use, with Particular Reference to Condoms

In view of the important role that condoms can play in preventing HIV infection, a section was devoted to questions about familiarity with, and use of, condoms. Respondents' familiarity with various contraceptive methods and their ideas on AIDS prevention were explored so that their experience with and attitudes to condoms could be viewed in a broad perspective and any misconceptions identified. Some of these items sought to elicit information on the perceived attributes of condoms.

Partner Relations Instrument

Marriage and Parenthood

An essential starting point in any investigation of sexual behaviour is to enquire about marriage or the existence of a regular sexual partner. The key items of information collected by the survey concerned current status and type of relationship (whether co-habiting and monogamous); length of current marriage/partnership; age at first 'marriage'; total number of current partners; date of most recent childbirth and total number of living children.

Contraceptive Knowledge and Use, with Particular Reference to Condoms

Knowledge of, and propensity to use, condoms is best interpreted within the broader context of family planning. Accordingly, knowledge and use of all major methods of contraception was measured, together with more detailed information about condom use. Condom use was studied in the context of commercial sex over the previous twelve months; sex with spouse or regular partner in the last four weeks; sex with non-regular partners in the last four weeks. In each case, regularity of condom use was established. Because the promotion of condom use is often hindered by adverse opinions about condoms, a series of questions was included on perceived attributes of the condom and condom use, as in the KABP questionnaire.

Heterosexual Behaviour

Heterosexual behaviour is of central interest. Although the range of information ideally required is wide, in practice the amount of data that can be collected on this subject is limited by respondent fatigue, recall ability, and, to a varying extent, by a culturally defined reticence to talk about personal sexual behaviour. The approach adopted in the PR surveys was to enquire about sexual behaviour in three different, albeit interrelated ways: namely, first sexual experience; behaviour over the previous 12 months; and behaviour in the last four weeks. The circumstances surrounding the first sexual experience were thought to be of particular importance in determining subsequent sexual careers. The main items of interest here were age at first intercourse, prior familiarity with the first partner; and whether that first partner was, or became, the spouse or regular partner. The collection of certain data over a 12-month reference period was considered necessary for two reasons. First, there might be seasonal variations in behaviour which reflected patterns of temporary migration or other social factors. Total reliance on a shorter retrospective span of time might fail to yield a comprehensive picture. Second, some forms of high risk sexual behaviour, in particular those related to sex involving payment or the exchange of goods, might be sufficiently uncommon as to be missed if questions were constrained to a short period of time. The main variables proposed for the 12-month reference period were number of non-regular partners, opinions on whether spouse has had non-regular partners, and the occurrence of sex for payment or the exchange of goods. More detailed information was collected for a four-week reference period because recall should be less of a problem. In addition to number of non-regular partners, information was sought on the frequency of sexual intercourse (both with regular and with other partners), marital status of non-regular partners, and on whether these partners were perceived to be sexually active with others.

Sexually Transmitted Diseases

The presence of certain other sexually transmitted diseases (STD) increases the risk of sexual transmission of HIV, and thus prompt recognition and treatment may retard the spread of HIV. Accordingly, a series of questions was included on the incidence of STD symptoms in the previous twelve months (or the lifetime incidence of STDs); treatment; and knowledge of preventive practices.

Knowledge, Attitudes and Beliefs about HIV/AIDS

This topic constituted the central concern of the KABP surveys. In the PR questionnaire, a subset of items was included. These included knowledge about HIV and its mode of transmission; perceived risk of becoming infected; belief that HIV can be prevented by behavioural change, and the nature of the changes either already made or intended.

For both KABP and PR surveys, additional optional sections were suggested. They included sections dealing with safer sex practices, medically related injection practices, locus of control, injecting drug use, and drinking habits. The purpose of these optional modules was to allow local research teams to expand the substantive content of surveys, where specific topics appeared to be particularly relevant. Thus they allowed flexibility without imposing a very lengthy instrument in all research studies.

Characteristics of the Surveys Selected for Comparative Analysis

In this volume, we do not attempt the herculean task of reviewing all the AIDS-related KABP and PR studies supported by WHO/GPA. Rather, the intention is to present the main results and implications of some of the better surveys on this topic in the developing world. The surveys selected were carried out in 1989 and 1990 using WHO/GPA protocols. The main criteria used to select the surveys for inclusion in this report are: adherence to the design and content of the standard protocols developed by WHO/GPA; availability of clean and documented data files by mid-1992; and reasonably high quality of survey implementation in terms of sample design, response rate, supervision and fieldwork.

All 16 surveys considered here satisfy these criteria; most (11) come from Africa, four are from Asia and one from South America. Tanzania conducted a KABP and a PR survey, and data from both have been used here. Hence, a total of 15, not 16, populations are represented.

At the time of the surveys, most of the countries represented had already established a National AIDS Programme and had started to launch mass media campaigns about AIDS. Typically, they had developed a one-year Short Term Plan and were in the process of developing a three-year Medium Term Plan. In most of the 15 countries, the surveys considered in this volume formed a component of these plans and were extensively used for the development of policies and activities.

At this period the status of the HIV/AIDS epidemic varied considerably between the 15 countries. In some cases, the epidemic was at a very early stage. For instance at the time of the surveys, only five AIDS cases had been identified in Mauritius, 39 in Togo, and less than 25 in the Philippines and Thailand. In contrast, 3647 AIDS cases were reported by early 1990 in Côte d'Ivoire, and the seriousness of the situation had been recognized in Kenya, Zambia, Tanzania and Rio de Janeiro.

Most of the principal investigators were senior social scientists or medical doctors belonging to major research institutions in their country. Some of them were closely involved in the National AIDS Programme. Two of them were even heading their National Programme, while others now have key positions in their National AIDS Programme. They developed their respective surveys with a local team generally funded by the government and the National AIDS Programme. Additional financial support to their institutions was usually provided by WHO/GPA. Technical assistance was provided occasionally to the survey team by WHO/GPA staff or consultants.

As already indicated, several protocols were developed at WHO headquarters in Geneva to provide a comparative framework for survey investigations. Seven of the 16 studies conform to the KABP protocol, six are PR surveys and three used the combined PR/KABP questionnaire. The principal investigators adapted these generic protocols in terms of coverage, design and content.

The WHO/GPA protocols provided recommendations for the design of the sample and its size. As a general rule, national probability samples of the general population aged 15 to 49 (or 59) were recommended. It was further suggested that sample sizes of 1000 to 3000 men and women were appropriate. All sixteen samples were selected on probability principles with various designs depending of the nature of the sampling frame in each country. A two-stage sample was generally used, with census enumeration areas as the first stage and households as the second. In some surveys an individual was randomly selected within the household. Typically, the responsibility for sample design was taken by national statistical offices. As shown in Table 2.1, 12 surveys are nationally representative samples and four are representative of cities (Lusaka, Manila, Singapore and Rio de Janeiro). The size of the

Table 2.1: Background information on the surveys

Countries	Principal Investigator	Institution	Type of Surveys	Number of Variables	Fieldwork Period	Sampling Method	Sample Size	Observations
Central African Republic (CAR)	Dr P. Somsé	Programme National de Lutte contre le SIDA	KABP	257	Sept/Nov 1989	Random sample	2431	National
Côte d'Ivoire	Prof S. Dédy Prof G. Tapé	Université d'Abidjan ENS d'Abidjan	PR	238	October 1989	Random sample	3001	National
Guinea Bissau	Dr Marcos	CESTAS-Bologna	KABP	309	Aug/Sept 1990	Random sample	1297	National
Togo	Dr G. Awissi	Programme National de Lutte contre le SIDA [Lomé]	KABP	207	June/Aug 1989	Random sample	2332	National
Burundi	Prof N. Ndimurukundo	Programme National de Lutte contre le SIDA [Bujumbura]	KABP	213	Jan/April 1990	Random sample oversampling urban zones	2264	National
Kenya	Dr P. Onyango Dr P. Walji-Moloo	University of Nairobi University of Nairobi	KABP	329	July 1989/Feb 1990	Random sample oversampling urban zones	2967	All Kenya except North Eastern Province
Lesotho	Dr A. Lawson	WHO Consultant for the Ministry of Health National AIDS Control Programme [Lesotho]	KABP/PR	243	Aug/Sept 1989	Two stage probability sample	1582	National
Tanzania	Dr E. Muhondwa	Faculty of Medicine Dar-es-Salaam	KABP	259	1989-1990	Two stage probability	4084	National
Tanzania	Dr E. Muhondwa	Faculty of Medicine Dar-es-Salaam	PR	230	1989-1990	Two stage probability	4171	National
Lusaka (Zambia)	Prof A. Haworth Dr K. Kalumba	University of Zambia Dept. of Psychiatry	KABP/PR	316	End 1990	Two stage probability	1992	Urban

17

Table 2.1: (Continued)

Countries	Principal Investigator	Institution	Type of Surveys	Number of Variables	Fieldwork Period	Sampling Method	Sample Size	Observations
Mauritius	Dr C. Chan Kam	National AIDS Coordinator Ministry of Health	KABP	194	July/Aug 1989	Two stage probability	2463	National
Manila (Philippines)	Dr T.V. Tiglao	College of Public Health University of the Philippines	KABP/PR	265	1990	Random sample derived from a household sample	1617	Urban
Singapore	Prof Kok Lee Peng	National University of Singapore	PR	183	Aug/Oct 1989	Randomly selected in four districts	2115	Urban
Sri Lanka	Dr A.J. Weeramunda	University of Colombo	PR	174	Jan/Aug 1991	Two stage probability	3012	National
Thailand	Dr W. Sittitrai	Centre for AIDS Research and Education, Bangkok	PR	360	Mid 1990	Stratified Random Sample	2801	Buddhist national population
Rio de Janeiro (Brazil)	Dr R.G. Parker	Instituto de Medicina Social, State University of Rio de Janeiro	PR	251	July/Sept 1990	Two stage probability	1341	Urban sample

samples ranges from 1297 persons in Lesotho to 4171 in Tanzania (PR). The average sample size is 2467 persons of both sexes, aged 15 and more.

Depending on the protocol, the focus of the questionnaire was on knowledge, attitudes and beliefs about AIDS or on sexual behaviour, as discussed earlier. However, the substantive content of the KABP and PR instruments had a considerable overlap. The content of the 16 surveys is summarized in Table 2.2. All of them collected information on the background characteristics of individuals and studied knowledge of AIDS (with the exception of Côte d'Ivoire). Questions on the sources of information about AIDS were not included in Côte d'Ivoire, Tanzania (PR), Singapore, Sri Lanka, Thailand and Rio de Janeiro. Beliefs and behaviours related to AIDS were not studied in Singapore, Thailand and Rio de Janeiro. The section on knowledge and attitude to condoms was not included in Côte d'Ivoire, Tanzania (PR), Singapore, Thailand and Rio de Janeiro. All the PR surveys studied the circumstances of first sexual relations (with the exception of Lesotho and Sri Lanka), sexual relations in the last four weeks and in the last 12 months.

The optional module on symptoms and experience of STDs was included in all the PR surveys, with the exception of Sri Lanka. Other optional modules were taken by some surveys, either KABP or PR, as indicated in Table 2.2. On average the number of variables collected is 252, ranging from 174 in Sri Lanka to 360 in Thailand.

In adapting the questionnaire to local needs and conditions, most of the principal investigators translated the questionnaire into the national languages and/or the local languages in order to ensure that the meanings of the concepts and questions were better conveyed to each respondent. For instance, in Sri Lanka the questionnaire was translated into Sinhala and into Tamil, in Burundi into Kirundi, in Mauritius into Creole, while in Togo it was translated into many languages including Mina, Ewé, Kabyé and others.

After back-translating into the original language in order to ensure the accuracy of the translation, the questionnaires were then pre-tested on small samples. The main purpose of the pre-test was to ensure that all questions were easily understandable and answerable by respondents. Pre-tests also provided an opportunity to amend the content of the questionnaire (including the pre-coded response categories) in the light of comments and reactions from interviewees. Generally 50 to 100 trial interviews were performed in each site. For instance, in Côte d'Ivoire the number was 120 interviews, in Mauritius 60, and in Kenya 400.

After appropriate introduction and the establishment of rapport between interviewer and interviewee, most of the sensitive questions, such as those on sexual activities, did not pose major problems. Typically, they were maintained in the questionnaires after the pre-tests without substantial modification.

As a result of these processes of translation and pre-testing, standard protocols were adapted to local conditions. In so doing, the wording of the questions might be changed, their order amended and less often questions

Table 2.2: Scope of the surveys

Sections of the Standard Questionnaire	CAR	Côte d'Ivoire	Guinea Bissau	Togo	Burundi	Kenya	Lesotho	Tanzania KABP	Tanzania PR	Lusaka (Zambia)	Mauritius	Manila (Philippines)	Singapore	Sri Lanka	Thailand	Rio (Brazil)
Individual characteristics	×	×	×	×	×	×	×	×	×	×	×	×	×	×	×	×
Awareness of AIDS	×		×	×	×	×		×			×					
Knowledge of AIDS	×		×	×	×	×	×	×	×	×	×	×	×	×	×	×
Sources of information	×		×	×	×	×	×	×			×	×				
Beliefs attitude and behaviour	×	×	×	×	×	×	×	×	×	×	×	×				
Knowledge and attitude to condoms	×		×	×	×	±	×	×			×	×		±		
Partnership		×					×		×	×		×	×	×	×	×
First relations		×					×		×	×		×	×	×	×	×
Relations in the last 12 months									×	×		×	×	×	×	×
Relations in the last 4 weeks		×					×		×	×		×			×	×
Symptoms/experience of STD	×	×							×	×		×	×		×	×
Sexual practices	±		×	×	×	±			×	×	±			±	×	×
Injection practices	×	×	×		×				×		±	×				×
Drinking habits	×	×	×				×	×		×	±	×			×	×

× = section taken   ± = incomplete section

might be omitted. Such adaptation inevitably leads to variability between questionnaires, which has to be taken into consideration in any comparative analysis.

As most of the surveys are nationally representative, the organization and the management of fieldwork operations was a complex and demanding process requiring a degree of national mobilization and publicity. The fieldwork had to be preceded in each case by a number of administrative steps. It was necessary to get clearance and support from the Ministry of Health, the Ministry of the Interior and various other bodies, depending on local conditions. Typically, each regional or district authority had to be informed about the survey and had to approve it. These steps and official contacts were also necessary for the efficient implementation of the surveys. District officials helped by providing accommodation to interviewers, transport, local interpreters and so on.

Various ministries and national institutions provided support to the surveys in terms of vehicles or personnel. In Sri Lanka, for example, community level health staff, including 12 Public Health Nurses, 126 Family Health Workers and 8 Health Assistants, were employed temporarily as field staff. In Thailand experienced interviewers from the Institute of Population Studies at Mahidol University were used.

Each national research team was responsible for the selection and in-depth training of the interviewers. The standard protocol recommended a training period of one to two weeks in order to familiarize interviewers with HIV and AIDS, to explain the purpose and design of the questionnaire, and to instill the confidence to elicit information on sensitive topics. Derived from the research package provided by WHO/GPA, a manual of instructions was provided to each interviewer.

The fieldwork in the various countries occurred mainly in the second half of 1989 and in 1990, though the PR survey in Sri Lanka was conducted in 1991. The duration of the fieldwork varied from one month to eight months. In most cases, it took two to three months to complete. Typically, such fieldwork was performed by mobile teams of interviewers headed by a supervisor whose duties included quality control and practical arrangements for travel and accommodation. The process in the field was first to identify the selected area and, in most cases, to list all households. The next step was to list all the household members and to identify those eligible for detailed interview. A random procedure was established in the sample design to select one or a number of members to be interviewed individually. Finally, selected individuals were interviewed, wherever possible in privacy.

Matching the sex of the interviewer and the respondent was recommended, particularly for PR surveys. However, for practical reasons it was not always possible in the field to match the sex of the interviewers and the respondents at the household level. The key requirements to elicit information on sensitive issues are clear and honest information on the purposes and use of the survey and an explanation of the reasons for asking sensitive questions. The quality of the answers is probably linked to the calibre of the interviewers and their training and to the degree of confidence established. The overall impression is that questions on sexual activities do not pose more difficult problems than any other area of inquiry. Certainly the response rates were much higher than anticipated, at over 90 per cent in nearly all the African surveys. Few people refused to participate or terminated the interview after starting. It may therefore be concluded that, if well prepared and carefully implemented, such surveys in the developing world are not much different from any other demographic or health survey.

As in most large surveys, teams were faced with major difficulties in the field, such as accidents, impracticable routes, loss of questionnaires, selected locations that could not be found and so on. One of the duties of the supervisors was to find solutions to these practical problems and, on the whole, they were successful. No survey was terminated during fieldwork.

After the fieldwork, the questionnaires were edited at the central office in each country and then coded, data entered and processed. The coding of the open-ended questions was generally done directly on the questionnaires. The principle was to take 200 or so questionnaires and create a coding frame of the most frequent answers. Because of this, most of the open-ended questions are not directly comparable between surveys because the coding frames differ. Data entry strategies varied across surveys. Some teams used tools such as dBase. Others used computer packages, such as EPI-INFO™ or SPSS DE™, which combine edit and entry. Except in Guinea Bissau and Kenya, all the data processing was performed in country by local teams following the Data Management Manual and tabulation plan developed by WHO/GPA (WHO/GPA, 1991). Data tabulation was done with SPSS™, with the exception of Singapore where data were analyzed with SAS™.

The national teams took responsibility for writing and disseminating their survey reports. The data were then sent to WHO/GPA for further comparative analysis. All files were fully documented and transformed to SPSS/PC System Files to facilitate processing.

Table 2.3 highlights a number of key characteristics of respondents who were successfully interviewed. The sex and age structure of samples will be discussed in the next section where data quality is assessed. It can be seen that the majority of interviewees were currently married at the time of the survey. The proportions married tend to be particularly high in the African surveys, a reflection of relatively young marriage ages. Conversely, the proportions are low in three of the four Asian surveys because of late ages at first marriage. In terms of rural-urban composition, there is considerable variability. Four of the surveys are entirely urban in coverage. Among the others, the percentage of respondents living in cities or towns ranges from 20 per cent in Kenya to over 60 per cent in Tanzania. As discussed later, urban areas have been over-represented in some surveys, thus compromising claims of national representativeness. Disparities in the educational background of

Table 2.3: Socio-demographic characteristics of the samples

	CAR	Côte d'Ivoire	Guinea Bissau	Togo	Burundi	Kenya	Lesotho	Tanzania KABP	Tanzania PF	Lusaka (Zambia)	Mauritius	Manila (Philippines)	Singapore	Sri Lanka	Thailand	Rio (Brazil)
Sex																
Male	51.5	50.0	65.4	49.2	50.4	43.5	34.7	39.0	44.0	48.8	50.6	39.7	47.6	50.2	40.2	46.1
Female	48.5	50.0	34.6	50.8	49.6	56.5	65.3	61.0	56.0	51.2	49.4	60.3	52.4	49.8	59.8	53.9
Ages																
15–19	19.5	21.9	13.7	18.5	22.3	16.8	16.9	16.9	19.0	21.2	13.0	21.3	15.5	17.6	15.3	12.4
20–24	21.3	20.9	14.2	17.6	20.1	15.7	17.9	19.2	20.7	22.4	14.6	17.8	18.2	16.3	14.9	14.4
25–39	42.8	36.2	38.1	38.1	44.0	39.9	40.8	40.8	45.5	41.7	43.0	37.3	45.0	43.1	50.1	50.8
40–49	16.4	9.6	15.5	13.4	13.6	14.3	16.8	13.1	14.8	9.1	14.5	13.3	21.3	23.0	19.7	22.4
50+	/	11.4	18.5	12.4	/	13.2	7.6	10.0	/	5.6	14.9	9.8	/	/	/	/
Marital Status																
Currently married	78.4	77.2	78.5	76.0	66.8	67.5	80.2	67.9	66.7	71.2	62.1	54.0	52.6	57.9	65.5	67.6
Formerly married	5.5	6.4	4.6	5.5	3.3	6.1	3.0	8.2	4.7	6.8	5.4	5.2	2.0	2.7	5.3	5.7
Never married	16.2	16.3	16.9	18.5	29.9	26.4	16.8	23.9	28.6	22.0	32.5	40.8	45.4	39.4	29.1	26.6
Residence																
Urban	34.3	55.0	36.9	32.0	50.3	20.0	32.0	61.0	58.4	100	58.5	100	100	36.6	32.1	100
Rural	65.7	45.0	63.1	68.0	49.7	30.0	68.0	39.0	41.6	0	41.5	0	0	63.4	67.9	0
Education																
None	42.4	41.6	45.7	45.2	45.8	24.8	14.5	26.9	24.0	8.9	11.9	1.2	3.2	/	3.1	25.2
Primary	33.6	23.6	23.3	32.8	39.0	47.9	46.5	61.4	66.2	33.2	45.9	12.2	23.0	/	66.5	29.4
Secondary & higher	24.0	34.8	31.0	22.0	15.2	27.3	39.0	11.7	9.8	57.9	42.2	86.6	73.8	/	30.4	45.4
Sample size	2431	3001	1297	2332	2264	2967	1582	4084	4171	1992	2453	1617	2115	3012	2801	1341

respondents are even more marked than rural–urban composition. In Manila, Singapore, Thailand, Lusaka and Mauritius, an overwhelming majority of respondents had received some formal schooling. At the other extreme, over 40 per cent of persons interviewed in Burundi and the four West African surveys had never been to school.

Issues of Comparability

Cross-national research on almost any topic is fraught with potential problems that may undermine the confidence with which direct comparisons can be made. Such problems are exacerbated when the subject matter is sensitive and potentially embarrassing, as was the case with the surveys represented in this volume. A selection of examples is provided here to illustrate some of the issues that arise.

Sexual Terminology

A number of authors have pointed out the difficulties of asking questions regarding sexual activities, not only in terms of the obvious problems of embarrassment and privacy, but also in terms of the ambiguity of many sexual terms. For example, Coxon (1988) discusses the varied meanings of the phrase *sexual partner* which emerged from his research with gay men in the United Kingdom. Activities that might be socially regarded as constituting *sexual partnerships* may be associated with quite different patterns of sexual behaviour and probabilities of transmission of HIV.

The standard version of the KABP questionnaire referred throughout the relevant sections to *having sex with*. Example questions include *Altogether, how many different persons have you had sex with in the last 12 months?* and *Have you received or given anyone money or favours in return for sex in the last 12 months?* On the other hand, the Partner Relations standard questionnaire refers to having had sexual intercourse as, for example, in questions such as *Have you ever had sexual intercourse? IF NO, I mean have you ever had oral sex, anal sex or vaginal sex?*

Although it is probably fair to surmise that the vast majority of people would interpret these questions in similar ways, their different levels of specificity might lead, in some cases, to different interpretations. For instance, mutual masturbation might qualify as having sex with someone, but would not qualify under the category of having sexual intercourse with someone. These alternative interpretations represent a potential threat to comparative analysis of levels of risk behaviour between sites, particularly for younger people who have not yet reached a stage of relatively stable sexual activity.

This potential danger of imprecision of meaning becomes more serious when the standard items are translated into different languages. For example, in the questionnaires used in francophone countries in Africa, the phrase *rapport sexuel* was used. Again, such a phrase leaves open the possibility of different understandings; this is compounded in countries in which a range of local languages and dialects were used for the questionnaires. Clearly, languages will vary with regard to the nature of the available terminology to describe sexual activity; indeed, the precise nature of these variations and their relation to the general attitudes within cultures to sexual matters, in itself, would be a fascinating area for further research.

General Ambiguities

Quite apart from the alternative interpretations of different terms and phrases, there might also be alternative interpretations of the same terms and phrases. Thus, for example, the question which asked about the occurrence of sex in return for favours, gifts or money may convey a variety of meanings. A man who buys a young woman a range of presents over a period of time and also engages in regular sexual activity with her might not perceive (or might not wish to perceive) the relationship as falling into the same category as more traditional forms of commercial sex engagement. The woman, however, might be prepared to engage in sexual activity only because of the presents obtained. (To avoid accusations of sexism, it should be added that such discrepant perceptions might equally apply in the opposite direction.) Interpretations of this question may reflect the general acceptance of such practices in particular cultures, which is likely to influence the level of willingness to recognize a primarily gift-exchange relationship for what it is.

There are other examples of general ambiguities which might be expected to vary across (and within) cultures; these include the items relating to knowledge about AIDS. There is a very difficult dilemma in designing questions on this topic, since it is never clear how much knowledge can be assumed on the part of the respondents. For example, two of the standard items asked, *How do you think AIDS is transmitted?* and *Do you think a person can catch AIDS from someone who has this disease?* Strictly speaking, both questions use incorrect terminology, since AIDS is not *transmitted*, and neither can it be *caught*. Respondents with very good knowledge of the distinctions between HIV infection and AIDS might have given technically correct answers but yet be classified as having been incorrect. Similarly, a question such as *Do you think one can get AIDS by having sex with prostitutes?* really deserves the answer of 'it depends', rather than the YES which was regarded as being the correct response.

Framing of Questions

Amongst the more interesting aspects of the variation between countries arose in the framing of the items relating to sexual activity. Local investigators were encouraged to adapt the standard version of the protocol for local usage as they saw fit; some local cultural flavour appears in the ways this was done. Consider some examples relating to first ever intercourse. The standard version of the PR questionnaire asked, *How old were you when you had full sexual intercourse for the first time?*, before going on to ask about how long they had known the person, their sex and other details. In the Singapore study, this wording was followed almost exactly, although the word 'full' was omitted and the men's version of the questionnaire asked about intercourse with a woman, and vice versa. The Central African Republic version asked *A quel âge avez-vous rencontré votre premier petit ami(e)? (At what age did you meet your first boy/girl friend?)*, followed by *Après combien de temps avez-vous eu des rapports sexuels? (After how long did you have sexual relations?)*. The point to note is the almost taken-for-granted assumption that the respondents will have had sexual relations with their first boy/girl friend.

By contrast, consider the version used in Mauritius where the following question was posed to those respondents who had never been married nor had a regular partner. *Il arrive que des gens (y compris des jeunes ou étudiants) aient des relations sexuelles même s'ils n'ont jamais été mariés ni ont eu des partenaires réguliers. Avez-vous déjà eu des relations sexuelles? (It happens that some people (comprising young people or students) have sexual relations even though they have never been married or have a regular partner. Have you ever had sexual relations?)*. This phraseology almost defies respondents to admit to such indiscretions! Such alternative forms of wording reveal interesting aspects of cultural attitudes to sexual activity. More importantly, the willingness of respondents to report honestly their own behaviour may depend upon the precise phraseology of the question. Alternative forms of wording 'give permission' to people to a greater or lesser extent to report behaviours which are potentially embarrassing or socially undesirable.

Comparing Scales across Sites

Even in cases where items and scales used in the various sites were more or less identical, there are potential problems associated with comparability. Although the standard instruments were not designed specifically to test particular psychological models of behaviour change, some of the items do bear some relation to well-used variables in such models. Examples include, *Have you yourself ever known anyone who has had AIDS in this community or country?* and *What are the chances that you yourself might catch AIDS? Would you say that it is (four or five point scale ranging from Not likely . . . Good chance)?* Many factors will influence the ways in which such items are understood and answered between different sites, including the level and extent of media coverage, the stage of the epidemic in the country concerned, and so on. For these and other reasons, the anchor points of the scales cannot be assumed to be similar. These measures are valuable for use in national analyses (although there may be sub-cultural variations in interpretation) where their association with other variables can be explored, but comparison of their absolute values across sites is problematic.

Conclusions

None of these examples is given to discredit the surveys reported in this volume. The intention behind the discussion is simply to draw attention to the complexities involved in designing questionnaires; these are exacerbated when dealing with sensitive areas in which there is no agreed language, and even more so when cultural sensitivities need to be taken into account. Such problems with questionnaire-based surveys have been acknowledged for a considerable time, but we feel it necessary to repeat them here to encourage readers to exercise caution in their reading of the material. While the data obtained in these surveys represent a tentative first – and innovative – step along the path of understanding aspects of sexual behaviour on a global scale, they do need to be complemented by parallel studies using more specifically tailored and culturally sensitive instruments, and by the adoption of qualitative methods to explore the dynamics involved in considerably more detail.

Data Reliability and Validity

The discussion in pages 24–27 warns us that the merits of the analysis presented in this volume depend critically on the quality of responses to survey questions that concern intimate and potentially embarrassing aspects of informants' lives. Indeed, this issue of data quality has implications far beyond the studies reported here. Hitherto, empirical investigations of sexual behaviour by means of large representative surveys have been rare. The main exception has been demographic and adolescent health surveys, many of which have enquired about timing of first intercourse and coital frequency within the preceding few weeks; but very few surveys have enquired about sexual contacts outside of marriage or regular partnerships, or about the numbers of sexual associates. These are critically important factors for any assessment of risk behaviour in the context of HIV/AIDS and constitute a central element of the WHO/GPA surveys. The AIDS pandemic has brought to the fore the need to describe and understand human sexual behaviour in different socio-cultural contexts. There is an equally urgent need to monitor changes in sexual behaviour, in order that the impact of HIV prevention programmes may be assessed. The contribution of surveys to these priority objectives depends entirely on the reliability of information that they generate. Poor quality data might well do more harm than good. For instance, large socio-economic or regional differentials in data quality could be particularly harmful by misdirecting prevention campaigns. Similarly, changes over time in the quality of survey data might mask genuine trends in behaviour and thus mislead policymakers. Owing to its complex and personal nature, suspicions about the trustworthiness of information obtained from sexual behaviour surveys are widespread. This in turn undermines confidence in the ability of social scientists to guide and evaluate anti-AIDS campaigns. It is therefore crucial that the quality of data obtained from empirical studies be evaluated.

There is no simple, satisfactory way of validating survey data on sexual behaviour. In addition to the usual problems of definition and recall that may beset most large household surveys, the collection of information on sexual behaviour is further complicated by the sensitivity of the topic: to what extent are individuals willing to report details of past sexual behaviour? Specially designed field trials provide the best opportunity for assessment of data quality. Accordingly, WHO/GPA initiated in 1992 a series of field studies into data quality. A variety of approaches was used. These include test-retest methods of assessing response reliability, split-sample approaches designed to compare the reliability of data obtained by different measurement procedures, in-depth interviewing of sub-samples of survey respondents, and known-group validation techniques. Sites in Senegal, Nigeria, Guinea Bissau, Uganda, Zimbabwe and Manila were selected for these studies. Preliminary results are reasonably encouraging (Dare and Cleland, 1993). Thus far, there are few grounds for believing that survey data are seriously flawed. There is also a growing literature in industrialized countries on the reliability of sexual behaviour data (e.g. Catania, *et al.*, 1990; Wadsworth, *et al.*, 1993), but we cannot assume that their generally favourable conclusions apply to the surveys that constitute the subject of this volume.

The possibilities for *post facto* assessment of the quality of data obtained in sexual behaviour surveys are more limited. Moreover, such evaluative analyses are unlikely to be definitive. Nevertheless, we can seek answers to the following questions:

- Are the findings of the WHO/GPA surveys consistent with other independent sources of information?
- Are reports of men and women mutually consistent?
- Are responses of an individual internally consistent?
- Do the overall patterns of results, and interrelationships, appear plausible?

The first question can be answered only in relation to characteristics that are commonly collected in censuses and other surveys, such as age, sex, age at marriage, urban-rural residence and the like. In a smaller number of cases, information on condom knowledge and use can be compared. A verdict of consistency on these dimensions is reassuring but, of course, tells us little about the reliability of more sensitive information on sexual behaviour.

Questions two and three concern consistency at the aggregate level between men and women and at the individual level between responses given in different sections of the questionnaire. The detection of major inconsistencies signifies defects in the data, though it may be difficult to identify the source of error. Conversely, high levels of consistency enhance confidence in the trustworthiness of information without yielding solid proof of its validity.

The fourth question, relating to plausibility, will be addressed in subsequent chapters, as part of the substantive analysis. As an example, it is concluded in Chapter 6 that the data on behaviour change are implausible and should not be interpreted literally. Conversely, in Chapter 4, the proportions of women saying that they believe their regular partner has other sexual associates corresponds quite closely with the testimonies of men about their own sexual behaviour. In this instance, the pattern of results is plausible and our confidence in them is increased.

Aggregate Consistency with Independent Data Sources

One of the objectives of the KABP and PR surveys on sexual behaviour was to interview a representative sample of men and women. A comparison of estimates of socio-demographic characteristics from these surveys with similar estimates obtained from other independent sources of information provides some insight into their representativeness and the extent to which their findings can be extrapolated to the general adult population.

Table 2.4 presents a comparison of estimates of the percentage of population that resides in urban areas and the sex ratio. With the exception of the Central African Republic, WHO/GPA surveys in the remaining ten countries for which data are available, in particular Burundi, appear to be biased towards urban localities. Some of the difference may be definitional in origin, but it is probable that many WHO/GPA samples do over-represent urban residents. Extrapolation of results to the total population therefore should be cautious. A comparison of the sex ratio shows a striking disparity in the case of Guinea Bissau where males far exceed females – almost twice the number. In contrast, females tend to outnumber males in KABP or PR samples in Kenya, Manila, Tanzania, Lesotho and Thailand. In Lesotho, the low sex ratio recorded in the survey may be genuine because of large scale out-migration of men to South Africa. In the other four surveys, however, men are almost certainly under-represented. This is a common occurrence in household surveys, because men are more difficult to contact at home and may be less cooperative. The remaining surveys appear to be quite comparable with regards to sex composition.

The above disparities in the sex ratio are further reflected in the comparison of the age–sex structure from independent sources for 12 countries.

29

Table 2.4: *Comparison of percentage urban and sex ratio*

Country	Percentage Urban		Sex Ratio*	
	WHO	UN[1]	WHO	UN[1]
Central African Republic	34	47[2]	106	94
Côte d'Ivoire	55	40[2]	100	104
Guinea Bissau	37	20[2]	189	94
Togo	32	26[2]	97	98
Burundi	50	5	102	95
Kenya	20	16	77	99
Lesotho	32	20[2]	53	93
Tanzania (KABP)	61 ⎫	33[2]	64 ⎫	96
Tanzania (PR)	58 ⎭		79 ⎭	
Mauritius	59	42	102	99
Singapore	–	–	91	104
Sri Lanka	37	21	101	104
Thailand	32	17	67	100

* WHO estimates are based on sampled age range, usually 15–49; UN estimates refer to the whole population
[1] Source: *Demographic Year Book*, (United Nations, 1990a)
[2] Source: *World Population Prospects 1990*, (United Nations, 1990b)

Apart from Côte d'Ivoire and Togo, external data for the remaining ten countries come from the United Nations (1990a and b). Data for Côte d'Ivoire are obtained from the World Fertility Survey 1980–81 (Direction de la Statistique, 1984) and for Togo from the Demographic and Health Survey 1988 (URD-DHS, 1989). In the case of Guinea Bissau, males over the age of 25 years, in particular those between 30–34 years, are over-represented, whereas those between 15 and 19 years are under-represented. For Tanzania and Manila, relatively more women in the younger age groups aged 20 to 34 years in the former, and 15 to 29 years in the latter, were included. On the other hand, samples from Kenya and Thailand over-represent women in the 25 to 39 year age interval and under-represent men under 29 years of age. The age–sex profiles of samples from Burundi, Central African Republic, Sri Lanka, Mauritius, Côte d'Ivoire and Togo are comparable.

In summary, some KABP/PR surveys have an urban bias. Apart from some inconsistencies observed in the sex ratio and further reflected in the age-sex structure, especially for Guinea Bissau, most of the surveys appear to be fairly representative on these basic demographic dimensions.

Comparisons involving marital status are more contentious than those for age or sex, because the concept is more complex. The WHO/GPA surveys used a very broad definition of marriage, embracing all partnerships that had lasted twelve months or more. The United Nations data, used for comparison, are derived from a variety of sources, no doubt employing a range of definitions (United Nations, 1990a and b). Typically, censuses and demographic surveys include *de facto*, or consensual unions, as marriages. However, unlike WHO/GPA enquiries, they usually exclude informal, non-cohabiting relationships. Where the latter type of sexual partnership is com-

Table 2.5: Singulate mean age at marriage (SMAM)

| Country | Date of Census/Survey | | SMAM (at 50 years) | | | |
| | | | Males | | Females | |
	WHO	UN	WHO	UN	WHO	UN
Central African Republic	1989	1975	20.4	23.3	17.2[1]	18.4
Côte d'Ivoire	1989	1978	20.7	27.1	16.9[2]	18.9
Guinea Bissau	1990	1950	21.4	27.7	19.9	18.3
Togo	1989	1971	21.5	26.5	18.2	18.5
Burundi	1990	1987	23.4[2]	–	20.8	21.9
Kenya	1990	1979	24.0	25.5	21.2	20.3
Lesotho	1989	1977	20.5	26.3	17.1[3]	20.5
Tanzania (PR)	1989/90	1978	25.2	24.9	20.6	19.1
Mauritius	1989	1983	27.9	27.5	24.0	23.8
Singapore	1989	1980	28.3[4]	28.4	26.3[4]	26.2
Sri Lanka	1990/91	1981	28.5	27.9	25.8[4]	24.4
Thailand	1990	1980	24.9[4]	24.7	22.1[4]	22.7

SMAM at age. [1] 35 years
[2] 40 years
[3] 30 years
[4] 45 years

mon, we might expect WHO/GPA surveys to yield younger ages at marriage than the United Nations sources.

The comparison is shown in Table 2.5, in the form of a single summary measure of the timing of marriage, the singulate mean age at first marriage, or SMAM. SMAM is computed by summing the proportions never married across age groups up to age 50 years, and then adjusting for the proportion still never married at age 50. It represents the number of person-years lived in a single state among those who will eventually marry by age 50. In a setting where first marriage patterns are stable, this measure is equivalent to mean age at first marriage. In the present application, the summation has been truncated before age 50 in a number of WHO/GPA surveys, because of erratic fluctuations in the proportions single at higher ages.

A wide range of SMAMs emerge among both men and women. In most of these countries male and female SMAMs between the two data sets are similar. A few countries, notably Guinea Bissau, Lesotho, Côte d'Ivoire and Togo, display relatively low SMAMs amongst the men included in the WHO/GPA surveys. Interestingly though, such variations are not observed among females. A close scrutiny of per cent ever-married figures for the 15–19 year age group reveals that, when compared to the UN data, a substantially higher percentage of men canvassed in the WHO/GPA surveys in the remaining 12 countries are in some form of a regular partnership. The main exception is Thailand. The difference between the two sources of information is not so striking or unidirectional for women in the same age interval. By age 50 years, in almost all instances, well over 90 per cent of both, men and women, have been in a marital union. This holds true for both the UN and WHO data.

Table 2.6:   Knowledge and use of condoms among women (15–49 years)

Country	% ever heard		WHO	DHS	% ever use	
	WHO	DHS	DATE	DATE	WHO	DHS
Togo	47.1	37.1	1989	(1988)	5.4	3.9
Burundi	47.9	12.2	1990	(1987)	5.6	0.2
Kenya	59.8	53.4	1990	(1989)	6.4	9.4
Tanzania	69.4	51.3	1990	(1992)	8.4	3.6
Sri Lanka*	–	73.3	1991	(1987)	10.5	9.4
Thailand*	95.4	87.8	1990	(1987)	21.6	12.5
Lusaka	72.4	73.3	1990	(1992)	21.1	9.1

* Sri Lanka and Thailand data refer to ever use of condoms among ever-married women between the ages of 15 and 49 years.

In part, the differences might be caused by the fact that the UN estimates for these countries are based on data collected well over 10 years ago (40 years in the case of Guinea Bissau) and perhaps it is now more common or acceptable for younger people to enter into some form of regular partnership at an earlier age. Successive changes in the legal minimum age at marriage and the possibility that couples exaggerated ages at marriage in order to be in conformity with the law are sources of bias of unknown magnitude.

We turn now to the last type of aggregate consistency check, concerning condom knowledge and use. This part of the analysis can only be performed for seven WHO/GPA surveys. In each case, the independent source of information is an enquiry conducted under the auspices of the Demographic and Health Survey (DHS) project. In DHSs, women aged 15 to 49 years are asked a series of questions on contraceptive knowledge and use. They are first asked to declare spontaneously which methods they have heard of. Subsequently, a brief description of each main method not already mentioned is read out, and respondents are again asked whether they have heard of it. For each method known, women are asked whether they have ever used it.

The PR variant of the WHO/GPA surveys used a measurement procedure similar to that of the DHS. The KABP instrument, however, did not include a probe for knowledge of each method, but only for condoms. If respondents did not spontaneously declare knowledge of condoms, this method alone was briefly described and prompted knowledge was ascertained.

The results of the comparison are shown in Table 2.6. Interpretation is difficult not only because measurement procedures varied but because there is no exact synchronicity between the two sets of surveys. Unlike demographic characteristics, knowledge and use of condoms is subject to rapid changes, particularly under the influence of AIDS-prevention campaigns. This factor goes some way to explaining the common pattern that WHO/GPA estimates tend to be higher than DHS ones. However, it is unlikely to account for all the discrepancies. In Tanzania and Lusaka, the DHS surveys were conducted shortly after the WHO/GPA ones. Yet in both instances, reported condom knowledge and use is lower in the DHS. It seems likely that the focus of the

WHO/GPA interview, with its emphasis on sexual relationships outside regular partnerships, on disease prevention, and on condoms rather than other methods of family planning, results in higher reporting than the DHS-style of interview. We are unable to conclude which approach gives the more accurate figure. It is possible that a more general type of survey, like DHS, underestimates condom knowledge and use, particularly among women for whom the topic may be embarrassing. But it is equally plausible to argue that WHO/GPA surveys yield exaggerated claims of condom knowledge and use. This methodological issue is of great practical importance, because of the need to monitor changes in AIDS prevention behaviours by both types of survey.

Aggregate Consistency between Reporting of Men and Women

This section summarizes some of the key findings of a detailed evaluation of WHO/GPA survey data on sexual behaviour (Mamdani, *et al.*, 1991). Data sets from five countries are scrutinized: Central African Republic, Côte d'Ivoire, Mauritius, Togo and Singapore. While data sets from Central African Republic, Côte d'Ivoire and Singapore do include information on whether or not the regular partner has been interviewed, they do not provide the appropriate identification that would allow for the linking and comparison of responses by paired regular partners on specific sexual behaviours. The analysis is therefore restricted to aggregate comparisons for respondents whose regular partner was also interviewed.

Data sets from the remaining two countries – Mauritius and Togo – do not provide the required information on whether the regular partner has been interviewed or not. Similar numbers of married men and women have been surveyed in Mauritius and their current marital status is similar. It is therefore assumed that the spouse of most respondents has also been interviewed. In contrast, the sample from Togo includes relatively more women in regular partnerships than men, suggesting that some of the husbands or male partners have not been interviewed. Nonetheless, a limited number of aggregate male/female comparisons are made.

Comparisons of coital frequency in the last four weeks with the regular partner can be made for the three surveys that used the PR questionnaire. The results, shown in Figure 2.1, are encouraging. In Singapore, there is a close correspondence in the responses of men and women. There is a suggestion of heaping of responses on *twice* and *four* times, suggesting normative types of answer rather than accurate recall. Similar heaping has been reported for DHS enquiries (Blanc and Rutenberg, 1991). In Togo and Côte d'Ivoire, there is a remarkable similarity in the proportions of men and women who state that no sexual intercourse with the regular partner had occurred in the preceding four weeks. These proportions are much higher than in Singapore, even suspiciously high, but the clear consistency with

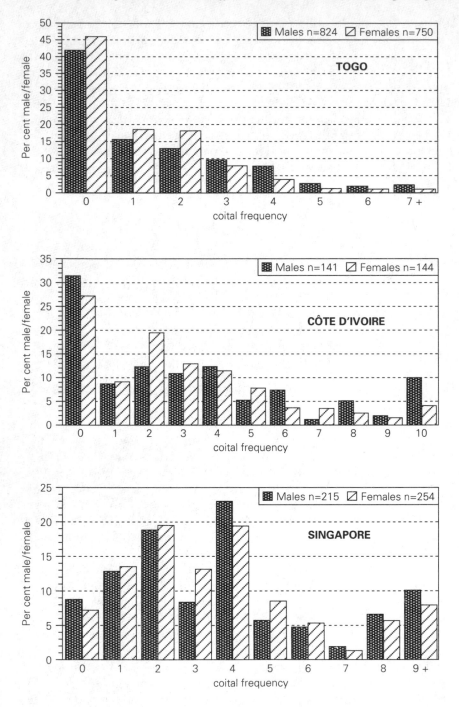

Figure 2.1:   Coital frequency with regular partner in the last four weeks

which both sexes have answered enhances their credibility. There is no evidence in any of the three surveys to support the commonly held view that men exaggerate coital frequency while women may underreport it.

For the same three surveys, a comparison was made of condom use with the regular partner in the last four weeks. In Singapore, where condoms are commonly used for family planning, men and women, on aggregate, gave almost identical answers; the percentages saying 'each time', 'sometimes' and 'never' differed by no more than one point. In Togo and Côte d'Ivoire, condom use within stable partnerships is rare; the answers of men and women are very similar, but this similarity largely reflects the very high level of negative responses.

Finally comparisons between men and women in reported number of living children were made for Singapore and Sri Lanka, but not for any African survey because of the confounding factor of polygyny. Aggregate male/female responses to total number of children are very close in Singapore and seem quite comparable in Mauritius, though a slightly higher percentage of the men reported not having any children at all in the latter survey. This may be due to the fact that, when the sample is limited to those currently in a union, the number of women exceed the number of men. It appears that some of the male partners were either excluded or did not respond to the relevant question. It is also possible that some of the women may be reporting on the number of children ever born rather than those alive at the time of the survey.

Tests of Internal Consistency

In this section, the focus is on the consistency of information supplied by individual respondents to different items in the questionnaire. In neither the KABP nor PR instrument were repeat or check questions deliberately introduced with an explicit aim of gauging consistency of response. Nor does the content of different sections of the questionnaires overlap sufficiently to allow a great deal of opportunistic, or *post facto*, consistency checking. Only three checks are possible for more than a minority of surveys. The first concerns reported age at first intercourse and age at formation of first regular partnership. When included, these two questions were asked in two independent sections of the questionnaire, typically separated by some ten to 15 minutes of interviewing questions. An alert interviewer or supervisor might have compared the pair of answers and enforced consistency by amending one of them, but the extent of such editing is impossible to ascertain. While inconsistency between the two items is suggestive of errors, the converse constitutes only weak evidence of there being consistency of response.

Cross-classifications of the two items were performed for eight surveys. The percentages providing inconsistent answers range from 0.1 per cent to

8 per cent. The mean level of inconsistency for men was 2.9 per cent and that for women 3.8 per cent. On this indicator of quality, the survey in Lusaka is least satisfactory, with inconsistency levels of 6.1 and 8.0 per cent for men and women, respectively. The next worst is the Côte d'Ivoire survey with corresponding inconsistency levels of 5.9 and 7.4 per cent. However, the overall impression is one of high consistency.

Two further checks were carried out. Both relate to the reporting of behavioural change in response to the threat of AIDS. First, a cross-check was made to ascertain whether respondents who claimed to have modified their sexual behaviour had shown an awareness of sexual transmission of HIV. Awareness of sexual transmission is generally very high, being close to 90 per cent among all respondents aware of AIDS. Among those who claimed to have modified their sexual behaviour, the mean level of awareness of sexual transmission is 96.5 per cent, among 14 surveys. Thus the mean level of inconsistent reporting is a rather trivial 3.5 per cent, and much of this may be attributed to errors in data management rather than respondent error. There is only one exception. In Sri Lanka, 14.5 per cent of those reporting a change in sexual behaviour had indicated a lack of awareness of sexual transmission in earlier questions.

A similar check was done for respondents who reported greater use of condoms in response to the threat of AIDS. There were only six surveys where 20 or more respondents gave this response. Unfortunately, among these respondents, the proportion who earlier said that they had never used condoms range from 25 to 35 per cent with a mean of 30 per cent. This makes inconsistent for this subgroup of the population the greater use and never use reports. This serves to confirm the interpretation in Chapter 6, namely that data on reported behavioural change should be regarded with scepticism.

Conclusions

This assessment of the quality of data obtained in the WHO/GPA surveys has been, of necessity, partial and rather superficial. The results have been mixed. The most disturbing disclosure has been the urban bias apparent in some of the surveys. This feature undermines claims to national representativeness, though weighting of data offers a partial solution. In a small number of surveys, there is also evidence of differential coverage of men and women that has led to deviations from expected sex ratios.

In other regards, the results have been encouraging. Age at marriage information is reasonably consistent with other sources, and the correspondence between men and women in reported coital frequency is impressive. Certainly, no gross errors of the type to vitiate substantive analyses have been detected.

Strategy of Analysis

Selection of Predictor Variables for Tabular Analysis

Individual country reports on the surveys conducted use a large variety of formats and many of the tables produced are not directly comparable. Accordingly, the general strategy adopted for this comparative analysis was to start again the process at the raw data level and to build fully comparable pieces of information. All the data were transformed to SPSS system files, and frequencies were run to assess variability between samples in the distribution of respondents across categories of key variables. Based on this initial data exploration, specific plans of comparative analysis were developed for each topic. A set of key predictors or explanatory factors was then selected for use in cross-tabulations of dependent variables. These predictors obviously had to be small in number, to be potentially powerful discriminants and to be measured in as many surveys as possible in the same format.

The section in both KABP and PR questionnaires on the background characteristics of respondents is the source of key socio-demographic predictors such as age, sex, level of education, urban-rural residence, religion and, in some countries, ethnic group. Some countries expanded this list with others. Though they are all potentially strong predictors of knowledge, attitudes or behaviours, some of them (for instance religion and ethnicity) are not amenable to cross-survey standardization and were therefore dropped. Those retained for the analysis are described briefly below and sample distributions may be seen in Table 2.3.

Current age of respondents was grouped as follows: 15–19, 20–24, 25–39, 40–49. These categories preserve the distinction between teenagers and young adults aged 20 to 24, many of whom are not yet married. There follows a broad grouping of persons aged 25 to 39. Finally the oldest cohort is distinguished on the grounds that their knowledge and behaviour may be distinctive. To maximize comparability, respondents over the age of 50 were dropped, because most samples had an upper age limit of 49 years.

Educational background of respondents was an automatic choice for use in comparative analysis. Exposure to schooling can be represented in the form of years of schooling variable or in terms of the highest type of school attended. The latter form was chosen, as not all surveys recorded the precise number of years of schooling. Because of the huge variation in the educational composition of samples (see Table 2.3), a coarse grouping (no schooling, primary, secondary or higher) was used.

For analyses of AIDS-related topics including sexual behaviour, marital status is another obvious explanatory or predictor variable. Marital status was defined in KABP and PR surveys in an unusually broad manner to encompass informal but relatively stable sexual partnerships as well as relationships that had been endorsed by legal, church or other ceremonies. The relevant questions in the measurement of marital status, represented by three categories (currently married, formerly married and never married), are:

- *Have you ever been married or had a regular partner? By regular partner I mean a person (a woman or man) with whom you have had sex for more than one year. She or he could also be someone with whom you have had sex for less than one year but with whom you intend to continue having sex.*
- *(IF YES) Are you now married or have a regular partner, or are you widowed, divorced or separated?*

From these questions, the definition of regular partner is clear. Any person with whom the respondent has had sex for more than one year (in reality or intention) is classified as a regular partner. Cohabitation is not necessarily implied. The characteristics of marriage and regular partnerships are discussed in detail in Chapter 4.

Another predictor directly relevant to analysis of knowledge and attitudes was based on exposure to three main mass media, newspapers, radio and television. For each of these media, the question took the following form:

- *During the past four weeks how many times have you read a newspaper (listened to the radio), (watched the TV)? Every day / Most days / At least once a week / Less often / Never.*

Answers were scored from 0 to 4 and summed for all three media. Total scores were then grouped into three categories: low, medium and high. The sample distributions are shown in Table 2.7.

The last predictor developed for the analysis refers to risk behaviour and is derived from several questions on sexual behaviour. From answers, two groups were formed: Some Risk Behaviour for those reporting that they had sex outside of marriage or a regular partnership in the last 12 months; and None or Limited Risk Behaviour for those reporting no sex at all in the last 12 months or no sex outside of marriage or regular partnerships. This predictor is documented further in Chapter 4.

Regression Modelling

Much of the analysis presented in this volume relies on simple frequencies and cross-tabulations which reveal the distribution of scores between, for example, different demographic groups. Whilst these are of great value, such analyses do not permit the determination of the relative contributions of particular explanatory or predictive factors to particular outcomes in a multivariate framework. Whilst there are a number of statistical modelling techniques which can be applied to data of the type collected in the WHO/

Table 2.7: Per cent distribution of respondents according to media exposure

Media Exposure	CAR	Côte d'Ivoire	Guinea Bissau	Togo	Burundi	Kenya	Lesotho	Tanzania KABP	Tanzania PR	Lusaka (Zambia)	Mauritius	Manila (Philippines)	Singapore	Sri Lanka	Thailand	Rio (Brazil)
Low and Not Stated	65.6	40.4	58.5	70.8	59.9	/	48.5	59.7	59.1	46.8	9.5	6.7	4.2	10.9	30.1	5.4
Medium	30.0	34.7	31.4	23.1	32.2	/	44.2	38.0	38.9	33.2	33.5	27.0	24.3	28.4	42.7	30.9
High	4.4	25.0	10.1	6.1	7.9	/	7.3	2.3	2.0	20.0	57.0	66.3	71.5	60.7	27.1	63.7

GPA surveys, the methods adopted here were multiple regression analysis (in the case of continuous outcome variables) and logistic regression analysis (in the case of dichotomous outcome variables). These methods permit the determination of the effect of each of the potential predictor variables while controlling for other variables (i.e. holding them constant). Thus, for example, where two variables each independently appear to correlate with a particular outcome when considered separately, including them in a multiple or logistic regression reveals which one (if not both) retains a relationship when the other is considered alongside it.

Building on the experiences of an earlier multivariate analysis (Ingham and Holmes, 1991), appropriate and interesting outcome measures and potential predictor variables were selected and regression models fitted to the data using appropriate statistical packages. All variables making a significant contribution ($p < 0.05$) in explaining variation in the outcome measure were identified and reported. Those non-significant are not reported. An advantage of this method in cross-national comparative analyses is that standard variables can be used (where the interview schedules allow) and comparisons made as to whether significant variables in one country are also found to be important in others. Should particular factors exert an important influence in a range of different countries (be they demographic or psychological variables) then greater confidence can be felt as regards the global importance of the implied explanatory relationships. Alternatively, divergent results encourage close consideration of features of particular countries which might help to explain the variation, and can lead to suggestions for different intervention programmes appropriate for different countries.

In addition to the variables described earlier, additional psychological and behavioural variables were used in the multivariate analyses. Wherever possible, similar variables were created from each data set to assist comparison. The technical details of the created variables are available in the original reports, which are available from WHO/GPA. In this section, the general details of the variables analysed are provided, together with brief reasons why they were selected and any recording that was necessary.

- *Perceived threat of AIDS:* the items relating to the extent to which respondents thought that AIDS was a threat to their country and/or community were combined to form a scale of perceived threat.
- *Perceived personal vulnerability:* the item concerning the extent to which respondents felt that AIDS was a threat to themselves personally was used as an index of perceived vulnerability.
- *Perceived severity:* the item relating to the proportion of people with AIDS who would eventually die was used as a score of the perceived severity of the condition.
- *Belief in asymptomatic transmission of HIV:* respondents were scored as positive if they indicated belief in the possibility of asymptomatic transmission on the relevant item.

- *Belief in sexual transmission of HIV:* respondents were scored as positive if they indicated belief in the possibility of sexual transmission on any of the relevant items relating to transmission of HIV through sexual contact.
- *Belief in casual transmission of HIV:* respondents were scored as positive if they indicated belief in the possibility of sexual transmission on any of the relevant items relating to transmission of HIV through casual contact.
- *Drinking habits:* respondents were classified as to the regularity of their reported drinking of alcohol.
- *Information exposure:* respondents were classified according to the extent of discussion of AIDS with family and/or friends, and/or exposure to AIDS information in the media.

The principle aims of the regression analyses are to search for patterns in the data of a number of types. In the first place, it is important to determine whether the demographic and socio-economic variables predict, in a systematic manner, the variation in various psychological and behavioural measures. This is important in that such relationships (if any) will assist in determining possible priority areas for .intervention with particular emphases.

Second, it is important to determine the extent to which, and the precise nature by which, the psychological and behavioural measures relate to each other. By modelling various relationships in the data, greater awareness is obtained as to the relative importance of particular variables, and, again, priorities for the nature and content of interventions can be determined. Thus, the demographic analyses help to determine who are the priority groups for intervention, whilst the psychological and behavioural analyses help to determine the content of such interventions.

Although formal psychological models could not be used precisely, some of the concepts identified in such models have been used to guide the analyses. Thus, for example, the Health Belief Model, developed in the 1970s by Becker and associates, identifies a number of variables which are relevant to the issue of health-related behaviour change, including perceived vulnerability, perceived severity, the costs and benefits of behaviour change, and reminders of the need for action (Becker, 1974). Later versions have added the concept of 'efficacy', or the extent to which individuals believe that behaviour change can actually lead to reduced probability of illness or disease (Rosenstock, Strecher and Becker, 1988). Clearly, some of the items in the KABP/PR questionnaires are directly relevant to these concepts, and are explored. Others, however, are not, so the Health Belief Model cannot be properly tested in its entirety.

A similar point can be made with regard to the Theory of Reasoned Action, developed by Fishbein and Ajzen in the 1970s (Fishbein and Ajzen, 1975), and recently amended (Ajzen and Fishbein, 1980). This approach points to the importance of two key concepts, attitudes and beliefs, on the one hand, and what are termed *subjective norms*, on the other. This latter concept refers to the extent to which important other people (for example, friends, parents, spouses) in the individual's social world would think about the individual performing particular actions. No items on the questionnaires could be used as a measure of this latter concept, although there are clearly various measures which can be used for the former concept. The Model, however, does stress the need to consider the relative contribution of these two areas; this is not possible with the present data sets.

However, although such formal models cannot be fully assessed, the concepts introduced in these approaches are still of great value. It can be argued that these concepts should be regarded as necessary conditions for behaviour change to occur, irrespective of their relative contribution in predicting actual behaviour change. Thus, the task of attempting to ascertain which, if any, factors can reliably be used to predict such concepts is an important one, and will help to propose directions for future research efforts more specifically designed to assess the relative value of the alternative psychological models available.

In order to confine the task of multivariate analysis to a reasonable size, two types of restriction were imposed. First, instead of analysing all 16 data sets, a sub-set of six surveys was selected for this aspect of the work. These are Côte d'Ivoire, Burundi, Lusaka, Manila, Thailand and Rio de Janeiro. The principle underlying this choice was to obtain a wide geographical representation of sites. The second restriction took the form of selecting only five key outcomes, or dependent variables, for multivariate investigation. These are: belief in casual transmission; risk behaviour; ever-use of condoms; perceived personal risk or vulnerability to HIV infection; and reported personal behaviour change. Naturally, the choice of predictor variables varies according to the nature of the outcome.

Chapter 3

AIDS: Knowledge, Awareness and Attitudes

Roger Ingham

Introduction

This chapter concerns levels of awareness of HIV and AIDS, the accuracy of specific areas of knowledge regarding transmission routes, the perceived severity of the condition, views on the appropriate ways in which to care for people who are HIV-positive, and attitudes towards testing. As already mentioned the information comes from surveys that were conducted in 1989 and 1990. No doubt, public knowledge and opinion has changed in recent years. Nevertheless, differences between countries, as well as the variations within countries, are of interest, and can still be used to assist the design of intervention efforts. Further, the baseline results reported in this chapter will enable the impact of such interventions to be monitored.

Clearly, awareness of HIV and AIDS is a necessary condition for behaviour change, although few would regard awareness *per se* as a sufficient condition. Whilst levels of awareness were generally high in most of the populations surveyed, there were appreciable intra-population variations in awareness. Perhaps not surprisingly, those respondents with lower levels of education and those with lower access to the media were less likely to have heard of AIDS.

General awareness of HIV and AIDS, of course, does not reveal anything about specific levels of knowledge. To assess the prospects for effective preventive behaviour change, it is crucial to ascertain views about the possible routes of transmission. A number of topics was covered in the standard questionnaires: knowledge regarding the possibility of infection by an asymptomatic person with HIV infection; the extent of erroneous beliefs about casual transmission (that is, through sharing utensils, clothes, etc.); and correct beliefs about transmission through unprotected sexual intercourse and sharing needles.

Ideally, of course, every individual should be able to discriminate effectively between potential routes as a guide to the adoption of specific forms of safer behaviour. False positive beliefs – for example, that HIV can be transmitted through sharing toilet seats – could lead to obsessively careful behaviour. More probably, such beliefs might engender a feeling of helplessness such that no changes are made simply because so many are thought to be needed. Similarly, inaccurate beliefs in transmission through purely social mechanisms are likely to lead to unwarranted discrimination and enforced isolation against those thought to be infected with HIV. Sex workers and homosexual and bisexual men will be particularly vulnerable to such discrimination, given the nature of much of the early publicity which accompanied the spread of the virus.

In general, accuracy of knowledge regarding sexual routes was very high, whereas accuracy regarding casual routes was considerably lower. In many countries, educational background and access to the media, not surprisingly, were good predictors of accuracy. Further items asked about the respondents' views on caring for people who are HIV-positive, or who have developed an AIDS-related illness. Respondents were asked who should care for people with AIDS (although the term *sufferers* was actually used on many of the surveys), where they should be cared for, who should pay for the care, and what should be done to prevent further transmission. Finally, the willingness of respondents to take an HIV test and related issues were ascertained. Opinions on these topics varied somewhat between countries, although substantial proportions in all countries expressed willingness to be tested.

Awareness and Knowledge

Awareness of AIDS

Most KABP questionnaires contained three items pertaining to awareness of AIDS. The first asked, *What do you think are the most serious diseases or health problems facing the world today?* followed by, *What do you think are the most serious diseases or health problems facing your country (or community) today?* Free responses were obtained, and, if AIDS had not been mentioned in answer to either of these two questions, then a direct question was asked, *Have you heard of a disease called AIDS (or local equivalent)?* Mention of AIDS in either of the first two questions, or a *yes* response to the third, is taken to indicate that the respondent is AIDS aware. (Analysis of the first two of these items is presented in Chapter 6.)

Table 3.1 shows levels of awareness among all respondents for all 15 study sites. Further breakdowns of levels of awareness for key sub-groups are given in Table 3.2 for those sites where the overall level of awareness was less than 95 per cent. Overall, the percentages of respondents who were AIDS aware at the time of the surveys ranged from 64 per cent in Togo to 99 per cent in Rio de Janeiro.

Generally, awareness in the francophone countries of central and west Africa was somewhat lower than elsewhere, with overall awareness levels of

Table 3.1: Percentage of all respondents who had heard of AIDS at the time of the surveys

Central African Republic	83.0
Côte d'Ivoire	89.8
Guinea Bissau	75.3
Togo	64.1
Burundi	96.0
Kenya	89.3
Lesotho	98.1
Tanzania	95.7
Lusaka	97.5
Mauritius	91.7
Manila	97.7
Singapore	95.4
Sri Lanka	76.9
Thailand	99.4
Rio de Janeiro	99.9

Table 3.2: Percentage of respondents who reported having heard of AIDS by background characteristics, for those sites where the overall level of AIDS awareness was lower than 95 per cent

	CAR	Côte d'Ivoire	Guinea Bissau	Togo	Kenya	Mauritius	Sri Lanka
Sex							
Male	87.4	93.9	77.1	72.6	90.1	95.2	79.2
Female	78.3	85.7	71.9	55.9	88.7	88.1	74.7
Age							
15–19	82.9	95.0	86.5	78.9	91.3	96.2	73.4
20–24	83.9	94.9	83.2	77.1	91.1	93.6	76.9
25–39	85.3	90.4	82.4	65.4	90.7	94.1	79.3
40–49	77.9	82.7	67.2	45.8	89.4	90.8	73.2
Education							
None	71.5	77.7	51.2	35.6	70.5	67.6	n/a
Primary	89.2	96.9	93.0	80.7	94.3	91.6	n/a
Secondary+	94.7	99.4	97.5	97.9	97.5	98.6	n/a
Marital Status							
Currently	82.4	89.1	72.4	60.5	90.0	91.1	75.6
Formerly	83.7	82.4	80.0	61.2	79.9	75.2	59.8
Never	85.8	95.7	87.7	79.8	89.7	95.5	80.0
Residence							
Urban	94.1	94.5	86.2	86.9	94.9	95.1	89.0
Rural	77.2	84.0	68.9	53.4	87.9	86.8	69.9
Media Exposure							
High	97.7	99.2	97.6	100	n/a	97.4	87.4
Medium	95.7	97.1	97.2	92.8	n/a	86.8	66.7
Low	76.3	77.6	60.8	51.7	n/a	74.9	45.1
Risk Behaviour							
Some	90.2	98.1	83.7	86.6	97.1	94.7	(84.8)
None	82.2	87.3	71.5	61.4	87.9	91.5	76.8

less than 90 per cent. The particularly low level of awareness in Togo was almost certainly related to the very high proportion of respondents in that country (71 per cent) who reported very low access to mass media. In all other sites at least 90 per cent were aware, with the exceptions of Kenya (89 per cent) and Sri Lanka (77 per cent). The extent to which respondents had heard of AIDS did not appear to be related to the reported prevalence of AIDS in the various sites (although the inaccuracy of prevalence data in most countries should be recognized).

In all populations, men showed greater awareness than did women, although the differences in the sites with high overall levels of awareness were minimal. The largest difference was found in Togo, where more males (72 per cent) than females (56 per cent) were AIDS aware.

Awareness in some African sites was lower among older than younger people. This age gradient may reflect the influence of level of education on awareness, since in most countries the old are less educated than the young. For example, in Togo, only 34 per cent of respondents who reported having received no education were AIDS aware, compared with 98 per cent of those who reported secondary or higher education. Similar, but smaller, effects of education were observed in the Central African Republic, Côte d'Ivoire, Guinea Bissau, Kenya, Mauritius and Singapore.

The reported level of media exposure (assessed by frequency of reading newspapers and/or listening to radio and/or watching television) had a positive impact on awareness in all settings, as would be expected, except in Thailand and Rio de Janeiro, both of which had very high overall rates of awareness. The proportions of AIDS aware respondents, according to levels of media exposure, are shown in Figure 3.1. Probably related to this factor was the effect of residence; rural respondents were less AIDS aware than urban residents (by at least 10 percentage points) in most of the surveys containing both urban and rural sites (the exceptions being Burundi, Kenya, Lesotho, Mauritius and Thailand).

Finally, cross tabulations of AIDS awareness with reported risk behaviour reveal that those who reported some level of risk tended to be more AIDS aware than those who did not, although, since risk is associated with age, this will again be confounded with age and marital status.

Logistic regressions were carried out on the data from four sites, with AIDS awareness as the outcome variable, and the demographic categories as the predictor variables. In three of the four countries (Central African Republic, Mauritius and Singapore) sex entered the best fit model as a significant predictor, with females in each case being less AIDS aware than males. Level of education entered the models in two countries – Central African Republic and Singapore – whilst marital status entered the models in Kenya and Singapore, with the previously married respondents being less AIDS aware. Interestingly, age did not enter any of the models, implying that it is indeed confounded with education level, and that it is the latter which is the more important predictor.

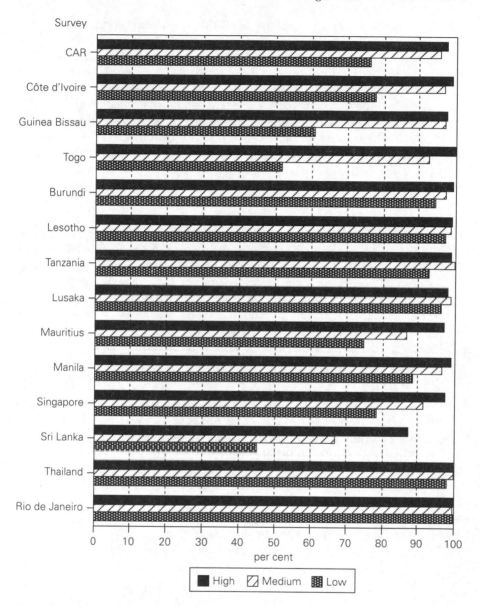

Figure 3.1: Percentage of respondents who have heard of AIDS, by level of media exposure

Specific Areas of Knowledge

Respondents who had heard of AIDS were asked a detailed series of questions regarding specific areas of knowledge and the routes of transmission. Identification of false levels of information amongst certain sectors of the population provides pointers as to the content and targeting of possible interventions to create the necessary (if not the sufficient) conditions for the need for change to be acknowledged.

Information on the prevalence and patterning of particular forms of knowledge is also useful in tracing the origins of such knowledge. Thus, for example, certain media may be consistently providing false information, certain myths may be particularly prevalent amongst particular groups and there may be a tendency for current campaigns to be persistently misunderstood. Detailed information on the possible origins of false knowledge can suggest corrective forms of intervention, such as encouraging media personnel to improve the accuracy and quality of their output. Those sites which used a PR instrument did not incorporate such a detailed section on knowledge.

The percentages given which relate to aspects of knowledge in specific areas throughout this chapter are based on the proportions of the samples who have heard of AIDS. This varies, as mentioned above, between countries. The corrected proportions for the overall samples can be readily calculated by adjusting the various figures provided by the 'AIDS aware' figures given in Table 3.1. For more detailed adjustments to categories within total populations, the proportions who have heard of AIDS disaggregated by demographic group are shown in Table 3.2 only for those sites where the overall proportions of AIDS aware respondents were less than 95 per cent. The actual proportions of the *total* samples thus included varies from 64 per cent in Togo to 99 per cent in Rio de Janeiro, as outlined above.

The questionnaires which did include the module on knowledge covered the following areas (with a *yes/no/don't know* response format):

- Whether someone who has the *AIDS virus* but looks healthy can transmit the virus to others (referred to here as *asymptomatic transmission*).
- Accuracy regarding a number of sexual transmission modes; although these varied to some extent across sites, most included items relating to potential transmission by *prostitutes*, having sex with a man or woman who *has the virus* (in some cases a distinction was made between use and non-use of condoms) and having sex with many people.
- Accuracy regarding casual routes of transmission. Again, the specific items varied across sites, but most included possible transmission by the following types of contact with someone who *has the virus* – touching, sharing food, sharing a room and kissing.
- Other topics covered included knowledge concerning possible transmission by being bitten by an insect (mosquito) which has fed on an AIDS sufferer, sharing needles, and whether it is possible for a mother to pass on the virus to her baby.

Knowledge of Asymptomatic Transmission

Accuracy of knowledge concerning asymptomatic transmission was derived from answers to the single item concerning whether a person who has the virus but looks healthy can transmit the virus. Respondents who answered *yes* were regarded as accurate, with the *no*s and the *don't know*s counting as inaccurate. Note that the item, in itself, does not distinguish between forms of transmission; thus, some respondents may answer *yes*, but under the false impression that it could be passed on by purely casual contact. The question is purely concerned with the possibility of asymptomatic transmission, and not the possible modes of such transmission. This item was not included in the instruments used in Côte d'Ivoire, Lesotho, Sri Lanka or Thailand.

Overall, the levels of accuracy fall within a fairly narrow range, from 71 per cent in Guinea Bissau to 88 per cent in Burundi (note that 33 per cent would be expected to be accurate by chance). There are no consistent variations between countries in different regions. This is an encouraging and perhaps surprising result, because the concept of asymptomatic infection, and infectivity, is an unusual one. The majority of infectious diseases are associated with visible symptoms. The acceptance by large majorities of these populations that the HIV virus can be transmitted by individuals who appear to be in good health represents a major achievement of information campaigns.

Levels of accuracy among men and women were reasonably similar, with the exception of Guinea Bissau, where there was a 14 per cent difference; 76 per cent of men were accurate as opposed to 62 per cent of women. In all other settings, the difference between males and females was less than ten per cent, the majority being in the direction of greater accuracy amongst men.

The effects of age were not consistent, although those in the youngest (15–19 years) and oldest (40–49 years) age groups were less accurate than others in the Central African Republic, Guinea Bissau and Rio de Janeiro; in Togo, Kenya, Tanzania and Singapore, accuracy was lower only among the older respondents. However, these age-related variations are small. Conversely, the effects of level of education were positive and pronounced in all countries. Thus, for example, in Guinea Bissau, Kenya and Mauritius, the difference between those with no schooling and those with secondary or higher was greater than 23 percentage points. Similar differences were observed in Singapore, although the absolute numbers who received no schooling were considerably lower. In all countries, the differences between those receiving primary and secondary schooling were also quite large, indicating a progressive increase in accuracy with increasing levels of schooling received. The single exception arises in Manila, where the very low number of respondents with no schooling – 16 people – record very high accuracy on this particular measure. These data are shown in Figure 3.2.

The level of media exposure also had a major impact on accuracy regarding asymptomatic transmission. In all countries, accuracy increased systematically with level of exposure, with the differences in percentage accuracy between the lowest and the highest levels varying from 26 points in Singapore to 13 points in Burundi and Rio de Janeiro. Similarly, area of residence

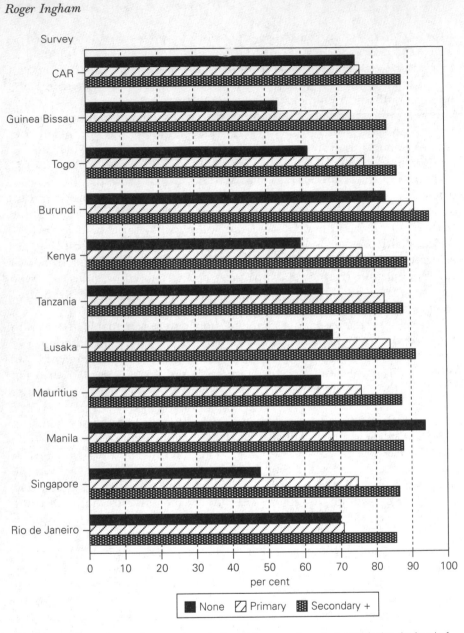

Figure 3.2: Percentage of respondents believing in asymptomatic transmission, by level of education

(where applicable) affected accuracy, with urban residents being between five and fifteen percentage points above rural residents.

Reported risk behaviours in the previous twelve months were associated with higher levels of accuracy in all countries except Singapore (in which little risk behaviour is reported). Given the finding that age was not consistently related to levels of accuracy, this would appear to be a direct relationship, not confounded with age. Those who reported risk behaviour were more accurate by between five (in Guinea Bissau) and 16 (in Kenya) percentage points.

Knowledge of Sexual Transmission

Accuracy regarding the possibility of transmission through sexual contact was defined by a correct response on one or more of the items (where included) which referred to the possibility of this mode of transmission (sex with prostitutes, having sex with many people, having sex with a man/woman who has the AIDS virus). Because the actual numbers of items used on the questionnaires in the various surveys differed, comparison between sites is not possible since scores based on random responses would produce different probabilities of accuracy (but see below for accuracy in specific areas). However, the intra-survey variations can be examined in an unbiased manner.

It is important to note that these questions, in nearly all cases, did not mention condoms; it could be the case that some respondents who were aware of the prophylactic role of condoms would have answered *don't know,* simply because this aspect was not clear.

Overall, accuracy was very high, with the majority of sites recording over 90 per cent accuracy, the exceptions being Sri Lanka (81 per cent) and Kenya (86 per cent). There was little variation according to the sex or age of the respondents, although older respondents in Côte d'Ivoire, Guinea Bissau and Kenya were slightly less accurate than younger respondents. Once again, level of education proved to be a major determinant; in all populations, those with no schooling were less accurate than those with secondary or higher schooling, the difference ranging from 3 per cent in Thailand to 20 per cent in Kenya, with the median difference being around 13–14 percentage points. Level of media exposure differentiated level of accuracy by more than ten percentage points (between high and low exposure) in Côte d'Ivoire, Guinea Bissau, Mauritius, Manila, Singapore and Sri Lanka, and urban residents generally showed marginally higher accuracy than did rural residents (an exception being Kenya). Marital status had little consistent relationship with accuracy regarding sexual transmission.

Reported risk behaviour showed a slight association with knowledge of sexual transmission, with those reporting risk during the previous 12 months having marginally higher accuracy scores in most countries. The largest of these differences (11 per cent) was found in Kenya, but in the majority of countries the difference between these groups was no more than three or four percentage points.

Knowledge of Casual Transmission

Knowledge regarding casual transmission was assessed by questions concerning HIV/AIDS transmission through purely social/casual forms of contact. The relevant items were *touching the body of, sharing food with, and wearing clothes worn by 'someone with the AIDS virus'*. As with sexual contact, direct comparison between populations is not possible since the actual numbers of items canvassed in the various sites differed. However, differences in accuracy between sub-groups are of relevance.

There were few consistent sex differences, although women in Côte d'Ivoire, Manila, Thailand and Rio de Janeiro were more likely than men (by more than ten per cent) to believe in the possibility of casual transmission. Older respondents were more likely to agree than younger respondents in the Central African Republic, Côte d'Ivoire, Manila and Singapore, as were those with lower levels of education in all countries except Lesotho and Mauritius. Levels of media exposure were also strongly related, with those least exposed to media being considerably more likely to believe in the possibility of casual transmission in all countries except Sri Lanka. No doubt related to this powerful influence of the media, rural residents expressed higher agreement than urban residents in all sites, again with the exception of Sri Lanka. Reported risk behaviour during the previous 12 months appeared to have an effect (by a difference of greater than ten per cent) in only three sites. Those reporting some risk behaviour were less likely to believe in the possibility of casual transmission in Côte d'Ivoire, Manila and Thailand.

It is important to note that fairly high levels of belief in casual transmission are not unique to developing country sites. Contemporaneous surveys in European countries and the US demonstrated similarly erroneous beliefs (for example, Blendon and Donelan, 1988; Hardy, 1990; Moatti, Dab and Pollak, 1992). Although there have been improvements in knowledge in these areas in some developed countries, these have only come to light as a result of repeated questionnaire based surveys. The improvements have been attributed to the introduction in such countries of national media campaigns amongst other factors (Stoller and Rutherford, 1989; Moatti, Dab and Pollak, 1992).

The existence of widespread beliefs in the possibility of casual transmission has also been found to be related to discriminatory attitudes against those who are infected with HIV (and/or thought to belong to a so-called *high risk group*), together with support for mandatory measures against such persons (Brorrson and Herlitz, 1988; Hogan, 1989; Rise, Kraft and Jakobsen,

Table 3.3: Among those who have heard of AIDS, the percentage whose responses were accurate on selected items

	PR	T	F	CL	M	MB	BL	N
CAR	93	60	54	38	26	78	87	85
Côte d'Ivoire	–	51	42	–	23	–	–	–
Guinea Bissau	89	69	45	36	22	71	86	82
Togo	92	40	20	19	11	80	90	82
Burundi	94	77	74	68	38	89	94	93
Kenya	78	75	64	–	51	68	82	80
Lesotho	93	67	53	–	–	86	81	84
Tanzania	92	66	53	42	41	81	90	86
Lusaka	77	88	–	–	–	88	–	60
Mauritius	92	49	24	39	30	83	92	87
Manila	68	76	–	–	–	82	–	–
Singapore	–	79	40	64	47	92	–	–
Sri Lanka	–	39	45	–	43	–	–	–
Thailand	–	63	44	–	30	–	–	–
Rio do Janeiro	–	93	43	–	43	–	–	99

Key: PR   Having sex with a prostitute
      T   Touching the body of SWA
      F   Sharing food/cooking utensils
      CL   Wearing clothes worn by SWA
      M   Mosquito bite
      MB From mother to baby
      BL   Blood transfusion
      N   Injection sharing needles

1991). Other researchers have, however, failed to find such relationships (Allard, 1989).

Knowledge of Specific Forms of Transmission

The accuracy indicators outlined above relate to categories of knowledge, specifically those relating to sexual and casual routes of transmission. Some examples of responses to specific items in these categories, as well as those in other areas of knowledge which were investigated in most of the countries, are shown in Table 3.3. Direct comparisons on all items across all sites are not possible since the actual items used varied according to the priorities of the local investigators.

Amongst the items relating to sexual activity, *sex with prostitutes* was seen as a possible route of transmission by around 90 per cent of respondents in all sites except Kenya, Lusaka and Manila, where the proportions were 78, 77 and 68 per cent respectively. Other items relating to the possibility of sexual transmission obtained similar scores, with, again, Kenya being rather lower than the others.

The questions on casual transmission were answered with much less accuracy, with some of these being near, or even below, the level which random responding would produce. Percentage levels of accuracy concerning *touching a person with AIDS* ranged from 39 per cent in Sri Lanka to 93 per cent in Rio de Janeiro. The accuracy of answers to *sharing food and/or cooking utensils with an 'AIDS sufferer'* ranged from 20 per cent in Togo to 74 per cent in Burundi, with the majority falling between 40 and 55 per cent. Accuracy in response to an item on *wearing clothes worn by an AIDS sufferer* ranged from 19 per cent in Togo to 68 per cent in Burundi, with three of the six countries that included this item falling between 36 and 39 per cent, close to the chance response level of 33 per cent. It is clear that Togolese adults in 1989 possess the least adequate knowledge about HIV/AIDS among the study populations. Not only is awareness of AIDS low, but among those aware, erroneous beliefs about transmission are common.

The item relating to risk *from mosquito (or other insect) bites* was generally answered with very low levels of accuracy, with scores ranging from 11 per cent in Togo to 51 per cent in Kenya. The majority of scores were below 33 per cent accuracy, indicating a worse than chance outcome. Accuracy of knowledge regarding the possible *transmission from an 'infected' mother to her baby* ranged from 71 per cent in Guinea Bissau to 92 per cent in Singapore, with the majority falling above 80 per cent accuracy. Similarly, *infection via blood transfusions* was accurately answered by more than 80 per cent of respondents in all study populations, as was the item relating to the possibility of transmission through *sharing needles for injections* (except in Lusaka). Recall that these items asked about the possibility (not the probability) of transmission through these routes, so agreement with the item regarding blood transfusions was scored as being correct, without necessarily implying that such forms of transmission are probable (which will depend on the policies regarding the screening of blood in the various countries). It appears from these results that information campaigns and other intervention activities can impart knowledge about genuine infection routes with some considerable success, but are much less effective at dispelling erroneous beliefs about transmission.

Regression modelling was carried out using the data from six countries (Côte d'Ivoire, Burundi, Lusaka, Manila, Thailand and Rio de Janeiro), with accuracy of knowledge regarding casual transmission as the outcome variable. This variable was selected since other areas of knowledge are reasonably high, and show relatively little variation within countries. Accuracy of knowledge regarding casual transmission, on the other hand, is fairly low in many countries. In view of the possible impact of such low levels of knowledge on preventive behaviour and on attitudes towards those living with AIDS, it is also of relevance to identify the factors which contribute to this situation. The predictor variables investigated were sex, age, marital status, level of education, urban/rural residence (where appropriate) and level of HIV/AIDS information exposure. This latter variable represents the extent to which respondents were exposed, through media coverage or discussion with friends and family, to HIV/AIDS information and/or discussion during the previous four weeks, and was only available in three of the six data sets

Table 3.4: Summary of regression models predicting belief in transmission of HIV through casual contact

Predictor Variable	Côte d'Ivoire	Burundi	Lusaka	Manila	Thailand	Rio de Janeiro
Sex	x	–	*	*	*	–
Age	–	*	–	*	*	–
Marital Status	–	*	*	–	–	–
Education	*	*	*	–	*	*
Residence	x	*	n	n	*	n
AIDS Information Exposure	n	*	*	*	n	n

Notes: * Enters models as main effect – (p < 0.005)
     x Enters models as interaction effect
     n Not available in country's data

from which regression models were created. The outcome variable was belief in one or more of the casual routes of transmission identified earlier (*touching the body of, wearing clothes worn by, and sharing cooking/eating utensils with someone with the AIDS virus*). The logistic regression results produced are summarized in Table 3.4.

It can be seen that age is a significant predictor in Burundi, Manila and Thailand, with the youngest and oldest age groups in each of these countries being less accurate (that is, more mistaken in their beliefs about casual transmission). Sex enters the models in three of the countries, with males being less accurate in Lusaka, but more accurate in Manila and Thailand. Men were also found to be more accurate than women in this regard in Haiti (Adrien, Cayemittes and Bergevin, 1993). Level of education is a significant predictor in five of the six countries (the exception being Manila), with the better educated in each case being more accurate. Of the three surveys covering both urban and rural residence, two (Burundi and Thailand) showed urban residents to be more accurate than rural residents, and the three surveys in which measures of HIV/AIDS information exposure were available all revealed that higher exposure predicted higher accuracy.

Beliefs about Severity

A number of items on the questionnaires measured the extent to which respondents regarded AIDS as an issue which directly affects themselves and others. This section considers some of these issues, whilst others are considered in Chapter 6. In this section, the degree of immediacy of the issue is assessed by the reported extent to which respondents heard something about AIDS on the radio, television and/or newspapers, and the extent to which they discussed the issue with their families and friends/colleagues during the previous four weeks. Second, the proportions who reported knowing someone with AIDS (SWA) are presented. Last, two dimensions of perceived severity are explored: the estimated proportions of those with AIDS who will eventually die of the disease, and the extent to which respondents believed that AIDS is curable. Chapter 6 will consider the reported general threat of AIDS to the world and country now and in the future, as well as the perceived personal vulnerability of the respondents.

The topics covered by these items are the same as some of the health behaviour change models developed by psychologists over recent decades. For example, the Health Belief Model (Maiman and Becker, 1974; Rosenstock, 1974; Rosenstock, *et al.*, 1988), which is probably the most widely adopted of its type, proposes that a number of factors predict the likelihood of behaviour change in a health preserving direction. Included amongst these factors are perceived personal threat, perceived severity, costs and benefits of behaviour change, and cues to action. Although the questionnaires used in the WHO/GPA studies were not designed specifically to test any particular psychological model, the analysis undertaken in this section will provide insights into some of the factors in these models.

At this juncture it should be pointed out that a number of writers have cast serious doubts on the individual cognitive approach adopted in such psychological models. Ingham (1994), for example, argues, amongst other matters, that the powerful impact of wider social contexts is relatively neglected and that reducing sexual decision-making to the level of the individual makes invisible many important social dynamics, including the role of power relations. Ingham and van Zessen (1994) propose that greater attention should be given to interactional processes. Other writers who have similarly questioned this general approach include Montgomery, *et al.* (1989); Pollak and Moatti (1989); Hingson, *et al.* (1990); Brown, DiClemente and Reynolds (1991); and Loewenstein and Furstenburg (1991). These latter authors remark 'like dieting, quitting smoking or arising early in the morning, sexual decision-making appears to involve more than a simple calculation of costs and benefits and dispassionate implementation of choice' (Loewenstein and Furstenberg, 1991: 963).

The reported extent of immediacy (similar to 'cues to action') of AIDS was assessed by three items, taking the general form: *Thinking back over the last four weeks, how many times would you say: (i) you have discussed AIDS with your family or relatives? (ii) you have heard or seen something about AIDS on radio/ television or in the newspapers? and (iii) you have discussed AIDS with your friends, colleagues or neighbours?* The response format ranged from *never* through *once or twice* to *more often*.

An item *Have you yourself ever known anyone who has had AIDS in this community or country?* was included, with *yes, no* and *don't know* being the response options. Again, this variable might be regarded as a further cue to action as proposed by the Health Belief Model; knowing someone affected may heighten awareness and perceived personal threat.

Perceived severity was assessed through two questions: the first was *Among the people who get AIDS, how many do you think will die of this disease?*, with

Table 3.5: *Mean aggregate scores relating to the extent of discussion of/exposure to HIV information during the previous four weeks (range 0–6)*

Guinea Bissau	2.39
Togo	1.32
Burundi	2.99
Kenya	3.03
Tanzania	2.30
Lusaka	3.25
Mauritius	1.37
Manila	2.60

response options ranging from *none*, through *some* to *most*, with a *don't know* option, whilst the second was *Do you think that a person who has AIDS or the AIDS virus can be cured?*, with response options of *yes*, *no* and *don't know*.

Extent of Exposure to AIDS Information and Discussion

The three items contributing to this scale were scored such that a response of *none* obtained zero points, *once or twice* obtained one point, with *more often* obtaining two points. The constructed scale for this variable therefore ranged from zero to six, with higher scores indicating greater discussion and/or information. This section of the questionnaire was not included in all of the surveys; the aggregate scores on these variables are shown in Table 3.5.

The mean scale scores ranged from 1.32 (in Togo) to 3.25 (in Lusaka). The former of these scores is consistent with results presented earlier, which indicated low awareness of AIDS in Togo, as well as generally poor levels of accuracy. There were some variations in the relative contributions of the different sources between study sites, as shown in Figure 3.3. Generally, coverage in the media was more frequent than was discussion with family or friends, other than in Burundi, where discussion amongst friends was slightly more frequent. It may be no coincidence that discussion with friends was most common among the four sites that are most affected by the pandemic (Burundi, Kenya, Tanzania and Lusaka). Discussions with families were not frequent in any country.

In all of the populations for which data are available, males reported higher levels of information exposure overall than did females; for example, in Togo, the mean score for males was 1.67 and, for females, 0.89, whilst in Burundi the respective mean scores were 3.41 and 2.57. Hearing of AIDS through the media was more frequently reported by males in all sites except Manila; similarly, discussion amongst friends was markedly more frequent amongst males than females.

The extent of overall exposure to information appears to rise with age up to the middle-age range, and then decrease somewhat. In particular, young people in Africa were relatively unlikely to have discussed AIDS within the family, and slightly less likely than older people to have discussed the

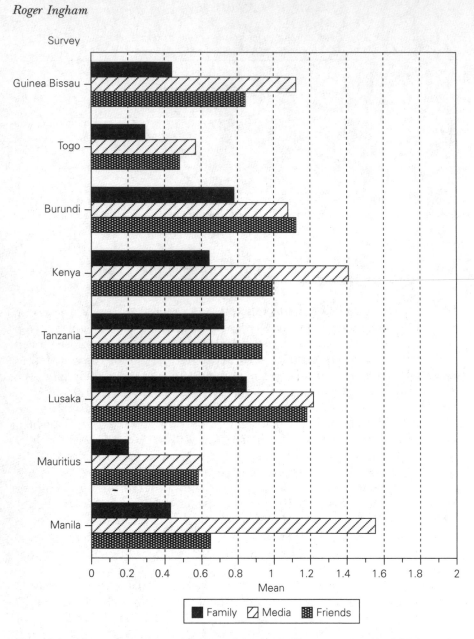

Figure 3.3: Mean scores of the relative contributions of different sources of AIDS information

matter with friends; however, there was little difference between age groups regarding information via the media.

Level of education had a major positive effect on exposure to all three separate sources of information in all sites except Manila (although the absolute number with no schooling in Manila is very low). Similarly, the level of media exposure had a large effect in all countries on all three dimensions; in other words, respondents who reported higher access to the media (newspapers and radio/television) reported considerably higher levels of discussion with family and friends. It is unclear, however, whether media exposure to AIDS stimulates discussion or whether there is a common cause for this association. Urban respondents reported higher discussion/exposure than rural respondents in all sites except Mauritius.

In sum, those who reported greater exposure to the issue of AIDS, through discussion with family and/or friends and/or through the media, were more likely to be male, living in urban areas, to have higher levels of media exposure and be better educated. Overall, the levels of exposure were considerably lower in Togo and Mauritius than in the other countries.

Proportions Who Report Knowing Someone with AIDS (SWA)

There are indications that the responses to this item may reflect ambiguities in understanding. For example, the absolute numbers of respondents who report knowing SWA in Mauritius is around 93, whereas at the time of the survey the actual number of known AIDS cases was five. It is difficult to believe that all of these 93 randomly selected members of the population knew these five people. This result suggests that the term *knowing* was interpreted rather widely, rather then being restricted to people known at a personal level. In other words, people *with AIDS* seen on television or elsewhere in the media might have been included in those deemed to be known.

Nevertheless, the overall percentages who report knowing SWA do hold some general interest; these are shown in Table 3.6. Those answering positively range from less than one per cent in Singapore to 57 per cent in Lusaka. As expected, the proportions are higher in the remaining African sites than elsewhere, with more than 11 per cent of respondents in the Central African Republic, Burundi, Lesotho and Tanzania reporting positively, followed by 4 to 7 per cent in the other African settings. In the non-African populations, apart from Rio de Janeiro, the highest proportion is 3 per cent in Thailand.

There are negligible sex differences in proportions knowing SWA, the largest difference being in the Central African Republic, with 27 per cent of females as compared with 18 per cent of males. Age has little effect on probability of knowing SWA, although in both Lusaka and Rio de Janeiro, older respondents are more likely to report knowing SWA. Level of education has a more marked effect in nearly all sites, with higher levels of education

Table 3.6: Among those who have heard of AIDS, the percentage who reported knowing someone with AIDS

Central African Republic	22.4
Côte d'Ivoire	7.1
Guinea Bissau	7.0
Togo	4.2
Burundi	11.2
Kenya	6.4
Lesotho	11.1
Tanzania	12.4
Lusaka	56.5
Mauritius	4.2
Manila	2.6
Singapore	0.7
Sri Lanka	1.8
Thailand	3.1
Rio de Janeiro	25.7

increasing the reported levels of knowing SWA. In the Central African Republic, for example, 31 per cent of the best educated report positively, as compared with 19 per cent of those with no schooling, whilst in Rio de Janeiro the respective figures are 34 and 18 per cent.

Level of exposure to the media also has a marked effect in most countries, with greater exposure leading to higher probabilities of knowing SWA. Similarly, urban residents are more likely to know SWA in most sites, the exceptions being Guinea Bissau, Togo, Lesotho and Mauritius. Those who report some level of risk behaviour during the previous twelve months are, if anything, more likely to report knowing SWA.

Perceived Severity of AIDS – Estimates of Curability and Mortality

Two items referred to the perceived severity of AIDS. Respondents were asked whether the condition was curable and to estimate the proportions of AIDS patients who, in their opinion, would die of the condition. These items were not included in all surveys. Results are shown in Table 3.7.

Belief that AIDS can be cured ranged from 3 per cent in Burundi and Tanzania to 29 per cent in Togo. The surveys in Mauritius and Manila each contained over 20 per cent of respondents who believed in a cure for AIDS, with Guinea Bissau and Lesotho each containing around 16 per cent. There were few variations according to sex of respondent; if anything, males tended to believe in a cure more than females, but the differences were not large. Opinion did not vary much by age, although in the Central African Republic, Lesotho and Lusaka younger people were less likely to believe in a cure than were older people.

Level of education of respondents has little consistent effect, although in Guinea Bissau there was a pronounced educational difference; 21 per cent

Table 3.7: Among those who have heard of AIDS, the percentage who believe that:
(a) AIDS is curable; (b) that 'most or all' people with AIDS will die of this condition

	(a)	(b)
Central African Republic	5	86
Guinea Bissau	16	36
Togo	29	66
Burundi	3	85
Kenya	5	–
Lesotho	17	–
Tanzania	3	73
Lusaka	7	85
Mauritius	25	72
Manila	20	81
Singapore	–	83

of those with no schooling believed in a cure compared with 11 per cent of those with secondary or higher level education. A slight trend in Kenya, however, pointed in the opposite direction. The level of media exposure had a modest effect in some countries, most notably in Guinea Bissau, where high exposure led to lower estimates of a cure being available (10 per cent with high levels, compared with 21 per cent for lower levels), and a similar gradient was obtained in Manila (18 compared with 29 per cent respectively). Data indicating a reverse relationship in Mauritius (that is, higher media exposure leading to less accurate responses) suggest that the content of media coverage of HIV and AIDS might warrant some attention in this country.

In sum, estimates of the extent to which AIDS is curable are rather high in some populations, possibly leading to false levels of security. In particular, Togo, Mauritius and Manila have over 20 per cent of respondents who are mistaken on this issue; on the other hand, accuracy is fairly high in the Central African Republic, Burundi, Kenya and Tanzania, where only 6 per cent or fewer of respondents are mistaken. Within study sites, there are few consistent variations between demographic groups.

For the second item relating to perceived severity, the proportions of those who reported that they thought *most* or *all* people with AIDS would die are provided. Note that the responses to this item are being used here solely as a measure of perceived severity; it would be inappropriate to interpret the responses as indicating levels of accuracy, since the official bio-medical estimates of likely life expectancy may well have varied across sites at the times that the surveys were conducted.

There appears to be little consistent regional variation in these data, with both the lowest and the highest overall proportions being obtained from francophone African countries. Women gave slightly lower estimates than men, although these differences were not large. There was little consistency in patterns with regard to age across the study populations. Level of education did make a substantial difference in all sites except the Central

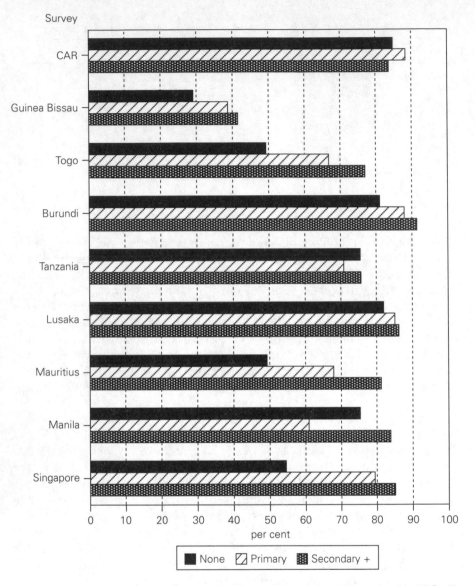

Figure 3.4: *Percentage of respondents who believe that 'most' or 'all' people with AIDS will die, by level of education*

African Republic, Tanzania and Lusaka (although the small number of those without schooling in Manila provided an exception to this trend). Educational differences are shown in Figure 3.4.

In general, higher exposure to the media was associated with higher estimates of mortality. However, there were interesting exceptions in Togo, where those with high exposure to the media provided lower estimates of mortality (59 per cent) than did those with medium (75 per cent) or low (74 per cent) exposure, and in the Central African Republic, Tanzania and Lusaka, where media exposure had no effect on estimates of mortality. Urban residents gave generally higher estimates than did rural residents, except in the Central African Republic, although none of these differences was more than a few percentage points.

Reported risk behaviour during the previous 12 months showed no consistent relationship with perceived fatality of HIV/AIDS, although in each of the surveys in which there was a difference of more than six percentage points, it was in the direction of greater mortality estimates being associated with some reported risk behaviour. This pattern suggests that estimates of the severity of AIDS do not affect levels of risk behaviour, although it should be remembered that the reported risk behaviour covered the previous 12 months, and there is a possibility that some respondents might have changed during this time period. Longitudinal research would be required to explore the nature of this relationship more fully.

In all sites, higher exposure to information and discussion regarding AIDS was associated with higher estimates of mortality. These differences ranged from around 5 percentage points in Manila to 15 percentage points in Mauritius, suggesting that higher exposure does lead to a more pessimistic perception of the severity of AIDS, although this variable is confounded with level of education received.

Finally, belief in the curability of AIDS was cross tabulated with perceived fatality of the condition. These data are shown in Figure 3.5. In all settings, large variations were found between these groups, with those who believe in the curability of AIDS also providing, not surprisingly, lower estimates of mortality. These differences ranged from 14 percentage points in Guinea Bissau (where the overall mortality estimates were low) to 40 percentage points in Burundi (where the overall mortality estimates were high). Although these differences are not surprising, it is of interest that substantial proportions of those who believed that AIDS is curable still believed that a large number of people with AIDS would die of the condition. These estimates ranged from 24 per cent in Guinea Bissau to 69 per cent in Manila, with each of the others being over 45 per cent.

Opinions on Caring for People with AIDS

Most of the questionnaires ascertained respondents' attitudes towards caring for people with AIDS, including the place at which they should be cared for, who should do the caring and who should pay for the care. Respondents were further asked what actions should be taken to avoid the risk of transmission by asymptomatic people with AIDS and the responsibility of the government for prevention. In terms of public acceptability of particular forms of action in the face of the threat and reality of AIDS, these are clearly important issues to consider.

Survey

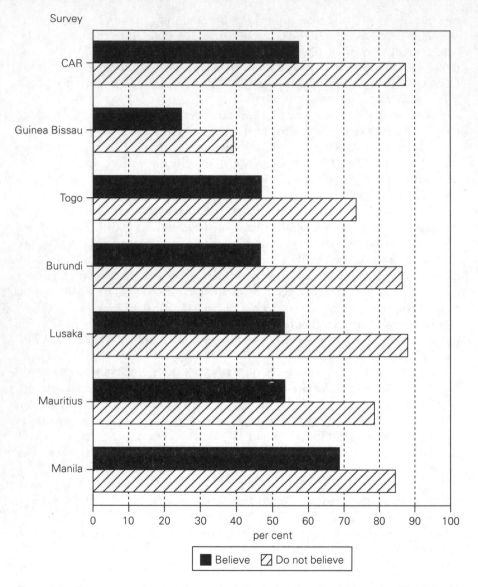

Figure 3.5:   *Percentage of respondents who believe that 'most' or 'all' people with AIDS will die, by belief in the curability of AIDS*

To the extent that government policies are responsive to the wishes of populations, the attitudes of citizens could have far reaching effects on the nature and quality of care provided for people living with HIV and/or AIDS. Further, it is now generally acknowledged that prejudice and discrimination against people with HIV have a real impact on the likelihood of spread of the virus (because people will not come forward for testing and counselling).

Investigation of such attitudes is thus of considerable importance to policy formation. Results from five questions are provided here:

1   *Suppose that a close friend or relative becomes ill and doctors decide that he/ she has AIDS. Where do you think he/she should be cared for?* The response options provided were *at home, general hospital, special hospital or clinic, don't know/other.*
2   *Who do you think should pay for the care and treatment of an AIDS patient?* The response options were *family (parents/children), charitable organizations, the government, don't know/other.*
3   *Who do you think should take care of a person with AIDS?* Response options were *his/her own family, ordinary doctors/nurses, doctors/nurses specially trained for this purpose, friends/other, religious or charitable organizations.* (In the Central African Republic, an additional option of *no care* was included.)
4   *Some people may have the AIDS virus and pass it on to other people without knowing about it. What do you think should be done to make sure that such infected individuals do not pass their disease on to other people?* Spontaneous responses were recorded by the interviewers for subsequent coding.
5   *Do you think the government should take steps to prevent the spread of AIDS? If YES, what are those steps?* This again adopted a free response format with subsequent coding.

None of these items was included in the questionnaires used in Côte d'Ivoire, Kenya, Lusaka, Manila, Sri Lanka, Thailand or Rio de Janeiro, and the following items were not asked in the countries indicated: (1), (3), (4) and (5) in Lesotho, (3) in Tanzania and items (1), (3) and (5) in Singapore.

Places for Care of People with AIDS (PWA)

For the six sites in which this item was asked, the frequencies with which each selection was chosen are shown in Figure 3.6. Respondents in three of the countries (Central African Republic, Togo and Burundi) stated a preference for general hospitals, whilst those in one (Guinea Bissau) preferred a special hospital. Caring at home was selected by a only small proportion of respondents, the highest being Burundi with 16 per cent selecting this option. In general, males expressed a preference for special hospitals, with females expressing a preference for general hospitals. The proportions of males and females selecting the home were similar.

Preferred Sources of Funding for People with AIDS

The results from this item are shown in Table 3.8. The majority of respondents in Guinea Bissau (52 per cent), Togo (83 per cent), Burundi (74 per cent) and Singapore (51 per cent) expressed the view that the *families* of

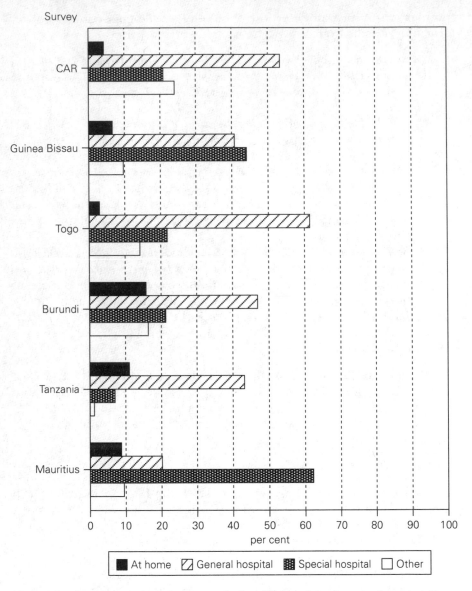

Survey

Figure 3.6: Percentage of respondents preferring different places for care of people with AIDS

people with AIDS should be expected to pay for the care of the patient; on the other hand, the majority in Mauritius (65 per cent) felt that the *government* should pay. *Charities* were cited by few respondents in each survey, while *other* was mentioned by 40 per cent of those in the Central African Republic. Given the coding of response options it is not possible to determine what is meant by this response (but see below).

Table 3.8: Among those who have heard of AIDS, the percentage of respondents choosing different sources of funding for the care of AIDS patients

Sources	CAR	Guinea Bissau	Togo	Burundi	Lesotho	Tanzania	Mauritius	Singapore
Family	48	52	83	74	74	52	29	51
Charity	4	8	1	1	–	1	2	3
Government	8	7	8	10	23	9	65	32
Other	41	7	8	15	4	36	3	14

There were few differences between men and women in preferred sources of finance, although in both Mauritius and Singapore higher proportions (12 and 21 percentage points difference respectively) of females felt that the family should pay, with correspondingly fewer preferring the government. On the other hand, in these same two countries, as well as in Guinea Bissau, increasing age was accompanied by increasing preferences for the government as the source of finance.

Preferred Carers for People with AIDS

The previous items asked for opinions on where people with AIDS should be cared for, and who should pay for this care. This item asked for opinions on who should actually carry out the caring. Percentages choosing *the family* ranged from 15 per cent in Mauritius to 52 per cent in Burundi; those selecting *normal doctor* ranged from 9 per cent in Mauritius to 27 per cent in Guinea Bissau, and *special doctor* ranged from 16 per cent in the Central African Republic to 74 per cent in Mauritius. These data are shown in Figure 3.7.

The category *no care*, included only in the Central African Republic, was selected by 39 per cent of respondents, higher than any other category. (Note that this probably accounts for the high number of *other* responses to the item on who should pay for care mentioned earlier.) This category is considered separately below.

There were few sex differences in these responses, although in both Burundi and Mauritius more females thought that the family should provide care, and more males preferred special doctors to general doctors in Togo, Burundi and Mauritius. Age made little difference to preferences, although there was a small non-significant trend towards preferring the family as age increased in the Central African Republic, Togo and Burundi. The category of *no care* in the Central African Republic was just as likely to be given by females as by males, was more likely to be selected by young people than older people (44 per cent of the youngest age group compared with 31 per cent of the oldest age group), by those with low media exposure, lower levels of education and in rural areas.

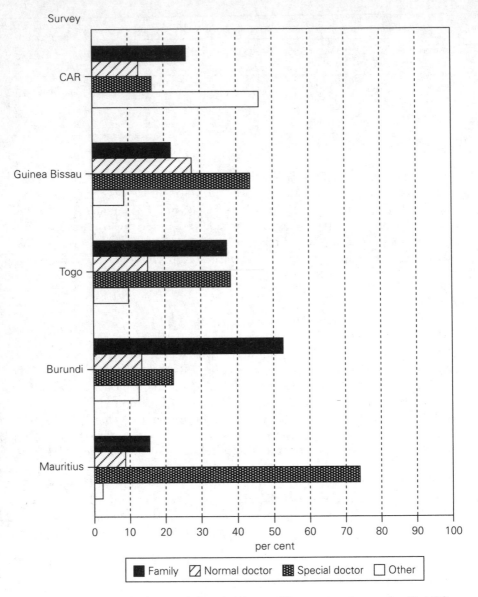

Figure 3.7: Percentage of respondents who choose different carers for people with AIDS

Preferred Policies to Prevent Transmission

Free responses were obtained to this item, so direct comparisons between surveys are not possible. However, some common categories were used in each country and these can be considered. The coding of response categories in the Central African Republic differed considerably from those used in the other sites. It should also be mentioned that in all countries the coded categories were not mutually exclusive, and their meanings are, in some cases, rather vague. A relatively high number of *other* responses were reported (ranging between 33 and 63 per cent), but it is not clear what is included under this heading in each of the surveys (in some cases, responses of *isolation* and *no idea* would be included under this heading). Despite these limitations, the data do provide a general picture of the predominant ways in which responses to the threat and reality of AIDS are prioritized.

Increased testing was a fairly common response, ranging from 41 per cent in Mauritius to 6 per cent in Guinea Bissau. Of course, testing on its own cannot be regarded as a prevention strategy, and it is not clear what was intended by those respondents who provided this answer. In some cases, selection of this option might have additionally implied isolation of those found to be HIV-positive, whereas in other cases it might have implied testing together with counselling. The frequency of selection of *education* ranged from 3 per cent in Guinea Bissau to 60 per cent in Singapore. Guinea Bissau also included the highest proportion of respondents selecting *measures to control sexual behaviour* as an option, with 18 per cent selecting this category. Variations between sub-groups were not large, although there was a trend for the better educated and those with higher media exposure to select increased testing as an option.

The responses in the Central African Republic included 15 per cent overall who believed that *killing* people with AIDS was the best means of preventing transmission, with a further 16 per cent advocating *isolation*. *Education and information provision* was selected by around 6 per cent of respondents, with sexual abstinence being advocated by a further 6 per cent. The category of *killing* was more frequently selected by those in the 20 to 24-year age group, the currently married, those with primary education and those in rural areas. High media exposure was associated with higher endorsement of *isolation* as an option. Reported risk behaviour did not affect patterns of responses on this item. It should be stressed that the coding of responses in the Central African Republic survey included the specific categories of *killing* and *isolation*, whereas the other surveys did not. These other surveys, however, did have rather large frequencies of *other* responses, and it could be that these punitive measures were included under this undefined heading. Thus, it would be inappropriate to interpret these data as necessarily indicating harsher beliefs in the Central African Republic than elsewhere.

State Responsibilities for Prevention

The responses to some extent overlapped with those of the earlier item, in that many of the means of prevention proposed in response to that item were regarded as the state's responsibility. Thus, dominant responses included *increased testing* (ranging from 4 per cent in Guinea Bissau to 19 per cent in Mauritius), *medical care* (ranging from 13 per cent in Mauritius to 54 per cent in Togo), *education/information* (ranging from 13 per cent in Togo to 26 per cent in Guinea Bissau) and *measures to control sexual behaviour* (ranging from 4 per cent in Burundi to 12 per cent in Togo). Although there were no strong discernible patterns of response according to demographic characteristics, it is of interest that increased *measures to control sexual behaviour* was more likely, in some sites, to be advocated by males, those reporting some risk behaviour, those with higher media exposure, with higher levels of education and in urban areas.

Again, the Central African Republic coding scheme included a rather longer list of options, with *killing* being mentioned by almost 22 per cent of respondents, and *isolation* by a further 24 per cent. *Killing* was more likely to be regarded as the state's responsibility by the younger respondents and those in rural areas, whereas *isolation* was preferred by older respondents, those with higher levels of education and greater exposure to the media.

Opinions on Testing

Attitudes towards HIV testing were explored in most of the surveys. If widespread testing were to be considered as an option as part of an HIV prevention strategy, then it is important to know something about acceptability, as well as the preferred mechanisms. However, there are some concerns over the usefulness of these data. First, no context was provided as to the possible implications of taking a test, whether it would be accompanied by appropriate counselling or would attract the kinds of punitive reactions mentioned above, and so on. Second, in some local contexts a negative response to this question could have implied fear or irresponsibility. Four items are considered in this section:

1 *Doctors can tell if you have the AIDS virus by carrying out a test on you. Would you be willing to take this test?* The response options were *yes, no* and *don't know/not sure.*

2 *Would you want to know the results of the test?*, with the same response options.

3 Respondents who indicated willingness to take a test were asked: *Would you want your family (i.e. your spouse, parents or children) to know the results of the test?*, again with the same response options.

4 Those who indicated a willingness to take the test and know the results were asked: *Would you tell them yourself or would you prefer someone else like your doctor to tell them?*, with *myself, doctor, don't know* and *other* as the response options.

These items were not included in the surveys conducted in Côte d'Ivoire, Kenya, Sri Lanka, Thailand or Rio de Janeiro, and items 3 and 4 were also omitted from the surveys in Lesotho, Lusaka and Manila.

The overall proportions who claimed to be willing to take a test ranged from 95 per cent in Togo to 67 per cent in Lusaka. Asian respondents were generally less favourably disposed to testing than African ones, with 69 and 75 per cent indicating willingness in Manila and Singapore respectively. In most of the African surveys (with the exception of Lusaka) over 87 per cent expressed willingness.

Males were more willing to be tested than females in Lusaka, Mauritius, Manila and Singapore, the differences being 9, 16, 11 and 14 percentage points, respectively. Age made little difference in most countries, although fewer of the youngest age group in Lusaka would be prepared to take a test, whereas fewer of the older respondents in Singapore indicated willingness. Proportions of those willing to be tested increased with higher levels of education in Lusaka, Mauritius, Manila and Singapore, and increased media exposure related to increased willingness in Mauritius and Singapore. Higher proportions of those who reported risk behaviour during the previous 12 months expressing willingness to be tested.

Very high proportions of those indicating willingness to take the test also indicated that they would like to know the result. The lowest proportions were obtained in Lesotho and Lusaka, with 89 per cent reporting *yes*; the other proportions were all above 95 per cent.

The majority of respondents overall reported that they would want their families to know the result of a test, the percentages ranging from 77 in Singapore to 95 in Togo, with the majority being above 86. Again, few demographic variations were obtained, although younger respondents and those reporting higher risk behaviour in Mauritius and Singapore would be *less* likely to want their families to know the outcome.

The majority of respondents in nearly all countries indicated a preference for informing their families of the test result themselves, rather than leaving it to doctors or other people. The proportions selecting *myself* ranged from 47 per cent in Tanzania to 84 per cent in Togo, with the remaining responses being *doctor* (as opposed to *don't know* or *other*) in nearly all cases. There were no variations due to sex, but a trend in some countries for younger respondents to prefer doctors to inform families. Other demographic variables had little effect.

Summary and Implications

There was some variation between study populations with regard to the proportions of people who had heard of AIDS, with overall figures varying from 64 to 99 per cent and a trend for lower figures in francophone countries in central and west Africa. Within populations, the groups least likely to have heard of AIDS were women, those with lower levels of education, those in rural, as opposed to urban, areas and those with lower media exposure. Such results suggest that attention needs to be directed towards devising means of informing these groups, perhaps through outreach and other community based approaches. Of course, such results also draw attention to the massive effect of structural factors on the potential for health amongst the population but, as in many such cases, interventions need to be devised on a considerably shorter timescale than that on which such structural improvements will be achieved.

Awareness in itself, however, does not lead to behaviour change to reduce risk. Specific knowledge regarding the virus and its routes of transmission are also essential prerequisites for change, albeit not sufficient prerequisites. Generally, levels of accuracy concerning actual routes of transmission (sexual, mother-to-baby, sharing injecting needles) were high. However, accuracy levels regarding transmission through casual routes were generally very poor, with some mean scores being below the level that would be expected by random answering of these items.

This is clearly an area which deserves urgent attention. The impact of such misinformation is potentially extremely serious, in terms of increasing general levels of anxiety, leading to a possible sense of helplessness (which may inhibit any change at all) and the likely discrimination against people known or thought to be HIV-positive. The specific content of campaigns and other forms of intervention needs to be carefully formulated to overcome such misapprehensions. Again, as was the case with AIDS awareness, accuracy levels were strongly associated with levels of education and access to the media. In a few countries, those with higher access to the media were actually less well informed than others. This suggests that the content of media coverage needs to be carefully considered, although it is difficult on the basis of the data collected in these surveys to ascertain whether such apparently misleading media coverage arises from official campaigns or more sensational features. Direct contact with reporters and editors may assist in reducing the probability of misleading information being presented, either intentionally or unintentionally.

The results for Kenya and Mauritius showed relatively lower levels of accuracy regarding sexual routes of transmission, although the Kenyan respondents were more accurate than those of the other countries regarding the (non-) possibility of casual transmission. Accuracy of knowledge regarding casual transmission was particularly low in Mauritius and Togo.

The level of education received emerged as a major predictor of overall knowledge, as did age, in some cases independently from education. Regression models constructed to predict belief in casual transmission in six countries showed that education had a major effect independently of other variables, and other demographic variables were each important in some, but not all, of the countries. Respondents who reported risk behaviour during the previous 12 months did not appear to be less well informed than others; indeed, the opposite was true in many areas. These findings confirm other work in demonstrating that knowledge *per se* does not lead to behaviour change in the direction of risk reduction. Similarly, estimates of AIDS fatality were no lower amongst those reporting risk behaviour.

Discussion of, and exposure to, information regarding HIV/AIDS was more commonly reported by males than by females in all countries, and higher exposure was also related to level of education and (not surprisingly) the extent of reported access to the media. The extent to which respondents reported knowing someone with AIDS varied quite considerably across countries, but there were no variations between subgroups of the populations.

There was particularly poor knowledge regarding the curability of AIDS in some countries; in half of the ten surveys in which this item was included, 15 per cent or more of the respondents held unduly optimistic beliefs. Level of education was the only factor which related fairly consistently to the probability of accuracy in this area. Similarly, estimates of the mortality of people with AIDS were particularly low in some countries, with only 36 per cent in Guinea Bissau believing that *most* or *all* will eventually die of the condition. Proportions in other settings ranged from 66 to 86 per cent. Again, educational status was associated with greater accuracy, as were media exposure and discussion about AIDS with friends and families.

Some caution needs to be exercised in interpreting the results regarding attitudes towards people living with HIV or AIDS. The different response options, and the ambiguity of some of the categories, makes it difficult to draw any firm conclusions regarding attitudes in these areas.

There did appear to be variations between sites in opinions on where people with AIDS should be cared for, who should pay and who should do the caring, although some of these variations may be related to differences in the health care systems in the countries concerned. The selection of the family as a major source of care and finance in some countries is of interest, given the demands that would be placed on family members through the adoption of such policies. With regard to the suggested strategies for the prevention of the spread of HIV, perhaps the most striking results were the generally low levels of support for education. The fairly high frequencies of selection of punitive and restrictive measures as a way of responding to the threat of HIV raises both ethical and pragmatic issues. In the former case, responses such as *isolation* or *killing* of people with AIDS are unwelcome, and may well be directly related to the levels of misinformation regarding transmission characteristics. From a more pragmatic position, such prejudice and discrimination will inhibit people who may be at risk from coming forward for testing and counselling, and may well lead to continued infections.

The policy implications are quite clear; the content of interventions (whether through the media or through direct contact, such as peer education, work with young people in schools and workplace discussion groups) needs to be considered in the light of these findings, and culturally specific and relevant means of overcoming such prejudice need to be devised.

Finally, although the issues relating to risk behaviour are more fully dealt with in a later chapter, it is worthy of note that there was no clear relation between levels of risk behaviour and accuracy of knowledge or perceived severity. Indeed, in many sites, the relation was the opposite of that which would be predicted by health behaviour models. In other words, those reporting risk behaviour often had more accurate knowledge regarding transmission routes, and higher estimates of severity, than those not reporting risk behaviours. These results reinforce the critiques of such cognitive approaches, and serve as powerful reminders that knowledge and threat, whilst probably essential for behaviour change to occur, are by no means sufficient.

Chapter 4

Sexual Behaviour

Michel Caraël

Introduction

The central purpose of this chapter is to describe and analyze sexual behaviour that may carry an elevated risk of HIV infection. The emphasis is thus on sexual behaviour outside of marriage or other regular partnerships, restricting attention to heterosexual partnerships for reasons mentioned earlier. However, to understand, or even to describe, non-regular sexual contacts we have to take into account the existence and nature of regular partnerships. Of course, marriage has been studied extensively by anthropologists, though typically in rather remote, homogenous communities. Anthropologists have viewed marriage as an institution that follows strict rules and performs well defined functions: regulates gender roles, defines offspring rules, legitimizes children, transfers succession rights and so on. Functionalists, such as Radcliffe-Brown and Forde (1987), regarded marriage as an institution that permits the creation of new family units, forms the basis for the kinship structure and ensures the continuity of the lineage. In their view, marriage was also an important guarantor of the permanence and continuity of the juridical-political system.

Structuralists, such as Lévi-Strauss (1949), changed the perspective in seeing marriage as the means for the universal exchange of women and as a mechanism by which patrilineal groups can make specific alliances. 'L'échange, phénomène total, est d'abord un échange total comprenant la nourriture, des objets fabriqués et cette catégorie des biens les plus précieux, les femmes' (Lévi-Strauss, 1949: 33).[1]

The neo-Marxist school, particularly Meillassoux (1975), underlined the economic determinants and functions of marriage and emphasized the domination that is perpetuated by the old over the young through control of women's reproduction.

Despite the many insights gained, a key limitation of most anthropological studies is to interpret marriage as an incarnation of theoretical principles. With a few notable exceptions (e.g. Parkin and Nyamwaya, 1987), anthropological theory has emphasized marriage as an element of stability, equilibrium and social harmony. Less explored has been the study of marriage from a perspective of sexuality and sexual behaviour. Certainly, demographers are interested in such customs as post-natal abstinence because of its relevance to fertility, but for most investigators, sexual behaviour was only of interest insofar as it formed part of courtship and marriage customs. Despite the fact that marriage is not usually the only option for sexuality, other expressions of sex were regarded typically as an ephemeral issue. It remains true, however, that in most societies, marriage is the pole around which sexual culture is organized and the dominant marriage system in a specific society usually shapes sexuality before, within and after marriage. Thus sexual behaviour outside of marriage is perhaps best investigated within the context of marriage customs.

The dearth of empirical studies that directly address sexual behaviours reflects a lack of interest from anthropologists (Vance, 1991). This is evident from reviews of the literature on human sexuality in sub-Saharan Africa (Standing and Kisseka, 1989; Larson, 1989; Caldwell, Caldwell and Quiggin, 1989; Caldwell, Orubuloye and Caldwell, 1992) and in Asia (Sittitrai and Barry, 1990) where most of evidence about sexuality is anecdotal.

The neglect is surprising because the perpetuation of multiple taboos, beliefs, rites such as female genital mutilation, and perceived punishments for transgression such as child illnesses or female sterility, show that the control of female sexuality is central to the culture of all societies. In short, there is no lack of information on sexual behaviour but rather a lack of interest in a domain that never appeared to be a legitimate topic of academic study in the eyes of anthropologists, with some prestigious exceptions such as Malinowski (1929) and Mead (1949).

From the perspective of sexuality, the first burning priority is not to construct a theoretical model of marriage. Rather it is to define and measure the different forms of cohabitation or informal relationships that coexist in specific societies and that organize patterns of sexual behaviour. The WHO/GPA surveys reported here are a first attempt in that direction. While there is often a tendency in the literature on HIV prevention to emphasize culture and insist on cultural values as a barrier to risk reduction, WHO/GPA surveys were intended to contribute to a better understanding of links between sexual behaviour and key factors such as age, gender, education, marital status and residence. An implicit expectation is that, as in other social fields such as reproduction, family planning or health-seeking behaviour, these key factors will influence sexual behaviour in similar ways across cultural boundaries.

A greater knowledge of sexual behaviour in different socio-cultural contexts should have important implications for designing and evaluating educational efforts to encourage self-protective behaviours. There is an urgent need to acquire more information concerning patterns of sexual behaviour and their determinants and to use this for local, regional and global AIDS programme development. Thus the advent of AIDS has transformed research priorities. Sexual activity outside of marital unions now has to be a focus of major interest. Moreover, quantitative information on the incidence, nature and circumstances of both regular and transient sexual liaisons is required. Only with these data can the future course of the disease be predicted, appropriate countermeasures devised and the achievements of programmes monitored.

The WHO/GPA sponsored collaborative programme of large scale surveys was designed to begin to remedy this gap in our knowledge. By themselves, survey data, removed as they are from their social and cultural context, cannot furnish satisfactory explanations of patterns of sexual behaviour. Only when linked to other, largely anthropological, bodies of knowledge, will deeper insights be possible. No start is made here on this task. A much more extensive mapping of sexual behaviour is needed before any such attempt can realistically be made. Demographers, with a long history of survey work, have reached the point when nuptiality and fertility regimes can be related to other aspects of social and economic organization (e.g. Lesthaeghe, 1989). It will be some years before a similarly rich and geographically diverse body of empirical data on sexual behaviour will be available.

As described in Chapter 2, two main questionnaires were designed for use among the general population. The most commonly used instrument, the KABP questionnaire, concentrates on knowledge, attitudes and beliefs about HIV/AIDS but also contains a limited number of questions on sexual behaviour as an optional module. The second instrument, the PR questionnaire, focuses more explicitly on sexual behaviour, though it also includes sections on knowledge and beliefs about AIDS. This duality explains why, in later tables and figures, the number of study populations will vary according to topic and its presence or absence in the questionnaires.

The main lines of enquiry included in PR questionnaires may be summarized as follows:

- initiation of intercourse (age, number of sexual partners before first marriage/partnership);
- characteristics of marriage/partnerships (current status, total number, age at first, whether current union is cohabiting and polygynous);
- sexual behaviour in the last 12 months (number of non-regular partners, relative frequency of commercial sex, use of condoms for commercial sex);
- sexual behaviour in the last 4 weeks (coital frequency and use of condoms with spouse/partner, number of non-regular partners, coital frequency and use of condoms).

The rationale for the content of the PR instrument is descriptive rather than theoretical. It is intended primarily to document the reported frequency of sexual behaviours that may carry a risk of HIV infection, in particular penetrative intercourse with sex workers or non-regular partners without the consistent use of condoms. It should be noted again that no attempt was made in the majority of surveys to measure intercourse between persons of the same sex, nor to distinguish between different types of penetrative intercourse.

The design of the PR questionnaire and the section about sexual behaviour in the KABP questionnaire faced two major problems of definition and measurement. The first concerned the distinction between marriage, other enduring partnerships and more ephemeral sexual relationships. Clearly, these distinctions are multi-dimensional, complex and often subtle. Any comprehensive classification would have to take into account not only the persistence over time of a relationship but also the associated expectations and obligations. An admittedly blunt and over-simplified solution was reached. Any sexual relationship that had lasted for a year or more (or was of more recent origin but was expected to continue for a year or more) was defined as a regular partnership, regardless of whether it involved cohabitation or had been sanctioned by law, religion or custom. The terms *marriage* and *regular partnership* will be used interchangeably to denote these types of relationship. All other relationships will be referred to as *non-regular* (that lasted for less than one year) or *commercial* sexual liaisons (that involved the exchange of money, gifts or favours in return for sex).

The second problem concerned the choice of reference periods for the collection of behavioural data. A single round survey offers no ideal solution to the dilemma that a very short reference period may maximize the accuracy of responses but affords very poor measurement, at the individual level, of relatively infrequent behaviours such as contact with sex workers. The additional complication of seasonality argued in favour of a 12-month reference period for the collection of some data, while a four-week reference was used for more detailed information on recent coital frequency.

Overshadowing these concerns is the additional problem of validity. Some social scientists doubt whether standardized surveys can yield valuable and valid data on sexual behaviour. Similar doubts were raised about family planning surveys 30 years ago but were later shown to be largely unfounded. Whether a similar verdict on sexual behaviour surveys will eventually be reached remains an open question. The preliminary assessment of data quality in Chapter 2 provided no major grounds for alarm. Nevertheless, the results presented in this chapter should be interpreted with caution and at times a degree of scepticism.

The organization of this chapter is as follows: first, sexual behaviour before marriage and among young people is considered. Interest then focuses on the formation of regular sexual partnerships and their characteristics. Finally, sexual behaviour outside of regular partnerships is discussed. Insights into the indirect determinants of these behaviours will be gained by examining variations in relation to social, economic, marital and community characteristics. But there is no attempt to assess underlying values and subjective meanings and thereby provide a more comprehensive understanding. No apology is intended here. An overriding need is to provide rather simple descriptions of sexual behaviours, to identify target groups, to monitor changes over time and to evaluate the effectiveness of interventions. Surveys have the potential to meet this need. Conversely they have limited potential to elucidate the cultural context of sexual behaviour. As mentioned earlier, complementary anthropological and other forms of more intensive study are required for any comprehensive understanding.

Premarital Sex

Information about early sexual activity is of obvious value in defining the onset of potential exposure to various type of risk, such as HIV/STDs and unwanted conceptions. Measurement of the proportion of men and women who ever experienced sexual intercourse is highly dependent upon the definition of *sexual experience* or *sexual activity*. In PR surveys, the question asked was *Have you ever had sexual intercourse?*, using a definition of sexual intercourse that included vaginal, oral or anal penetration between two individuals but that excluded mutual masturbation, intercrural sex and other forms of non-penetrative sex. In most African countries, the definition was straightforward and did not need any clarification. However, in some Asian countries where flirtation, mutual masturbation and courting is common and prolonged, respondents may consider themselves as sexually active even when no penetrative intercourse has occurred. In such settings, the definition had to be stated during the interview. Despite this caveat, the proportion who have had sexual intercourse is likely to be comparable cross-nationally.

For sexually experienced respondents, a retrospective question was then asked: *How old were you when you had sexual intercourse with a man (or a woman) for the first time?* Such retrospective reporting is subject to considerable memory lapse, particularly among older people for whom the event is remote. Accordingly, much of the analysis that follows is based primarily on current status data. Interpretive emphasis is placed on statements that describe a person's current situation with regard to sexual experience or marriage, or on reporting of recent events. In this way, recall errors are minimized.

Sexual Experience Among Young People

The initiation of sexual intercourse early in life is associated with enhanced risk of HIV and STD (Dixon-Mueller and Wasserheit, 1990), owing to its effect on length of sexual exposure, unless first sexual intercourse marks the beginning of a mutually monogamous relationship. Though there is as yet no systematic body of knowledge about the proportion of adolescents who are sexually active or about the number of relationships that occur before the first longstanding partnership, there is a growing number of empirical investigations on this topic.

Table 4.1: *Percentage of men and women aged 15–19 years who were never married and who reported sexual intercourse in the last 12 months*

Survey	Males per cent	Females per cent
Central African Republic	69	56
Côte d'Ivoire	43	28
Guinea Bissau	51	30
Togo	18	3
Burundi	10	3
Kenya	54	44
Lesotho	33	16
Tanzania	37	24
Lusaka	16	10
Manila	15	0
Singapore	3	0
Sri Lanka	1	0
Thailand	29	1
Rio de Janeiro	61	9

Table 4.1 compares proportions of *never-married* males and females aged 15–19 years who reported sexual intercourse in the last 12 months. There are huge differences between African countries, from less than 10 per cent in Burundi to 69 per cent in Guinea Bissau. On the basis of this evidence, sweeping generalizations about sexual behaviour in Africa are unwarranted. Moreover, the levels of male sexual activity are lower than those reported by Morris (1990) for eleven Latin American cities, where 12 to 25 per cent of females and 44 to 73 per cent of males aged 15–19 reported premarital sexual intercourse.

For all fourteen surveys, reported sexual experience among young males ranges from 1 to 69 per cent, and among young females, from 0 to 56 per cent. In all study populations, the level of sexual experience was much higher among young men than among young women, with a median value of 30 per cent for men but only 9 per cent for women. Where the difference between males and females is very great, as in Rio de Janeiro, Thailand or Manila, we may infer that young men seek out older women who are already sexually experienced, sex workers or same sex partners. Such a pattern may enhance the risk of HIV transmission if such sex is unprotected. Despite these exceptions, there is a significant correlation ($R = 0.82$; $p = 0.0004$) between levels of sexual experience among males and females (Figure 4.1).

The level of sexual activity among never-married females in the four Asian study population is negligible. This result reflects strong social sanctions against premarital intercourse for women. For instance, in Sri Lanka, failure of the bride to demonstrate evidence of virginity on first marital intercourse may result in dissolution of marriage (Basnayake, 1986). In most Asian countries, all types of sexual relations before marriage are condemned by religious teachings, by laws and by public opinion (Sarwono, 1983).

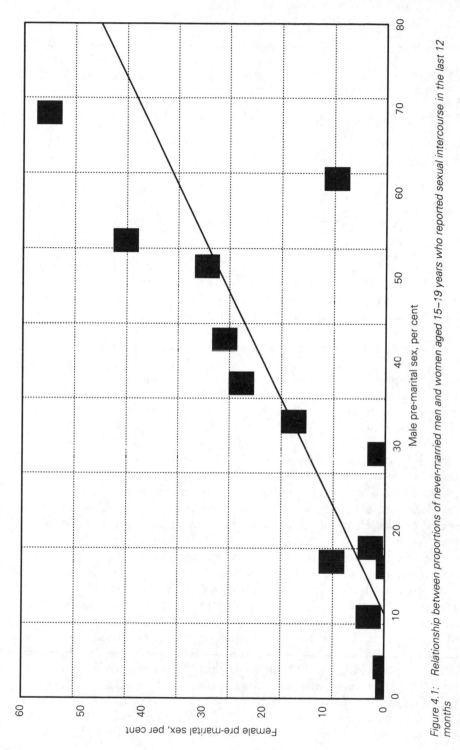

Figure 4.1: Relationship between proportions of never-married men and women aged 15–19 years who reported sexual intercourse in the last 12 months

Table 4.2: *Mean number of sexual partners in the last 12 months among never-married men and women aged 15–19 years*

Survey	Males		Females	
	All	Sexually Active	All	Sexually Active
Côte d'Ivoire	0.9	2.4	0.3	1.6
Guinea Bissau	0.6	1.7	0.5	1.9
Togo	0.2	2.0	0.0	1.0
Kenya	0.5	1.6	0.4	1.5
Lesotho	0.7	2.3	0.2	1.3
Tanzania	0.9	2.5	0.4	1.7
Manila	0.2	1.8	0.0	0.0
Singapore	0.1	4.5	0.0	0.0
Thailand	1.0	3.8	0.1	4.3
Rio de Janeiro	1.6	2.6	0.1	1.7

The rate of change in sexual partners among teenagers is often believed to be low because of the sporadic nature of their sexual activity. Data on the number of the sexual partners in the last 12 months show that this view is not necessarily true. The mean number of sexual partners in the last 12 months for never-married 15–19 year olds varies from 0.0 for females in Singapore and Manila to 1.6 for Rio de Janeiro males. Those reporting sexual intercourse in the last 12 months averaged from 1 to 4.5 partners. The highest mean numbers are found in Thailand and Singapore. These are both societies where few young unmarried women report sexual intercourse. Thus it appears likely that the large numbers of partners reported by sexually active men reflect contacts with sex workers. In all settings, males report higher number of partners than females. There are several explanations for the gender difference. Young males may have contacts with sex workers as is probably the case in Singapore and Thailand. Alternatively, males may have contacts with older females though this explanation is less plausible.

Cities are generally associated with less parental control of adolescent sexual behaviour, more social mixing and more exposure to modern life-styles (Caraël, 1987; Larson, 1989). For those surveys containing separate urban and rural domains, rural–urban comparisons of the proportions of unmarried male and female respondents aged 15 to 19 reporting sexual intercourse in the last 12 months are shown in Figure 4.2. The proportions are higher in urban than in rural settings in Togo, Burundi, Tanzania, Central African Republic and Sri Lanka. In the other surveys, however, initiation of sexual activity before marriage begins earlier in rural than in urban settings, or at the same time. These results reflect the relative importance attached to virginity in different traditions. They also show that an urban residence is not necessarily or always associated with greater sexual freedom for young people. Patterns of urbanization vary between countries and, accordingly, shape sexual culture differently. Rural–urban communication and circulation, seasonal migration, sex ratios in urban and rural settings, and

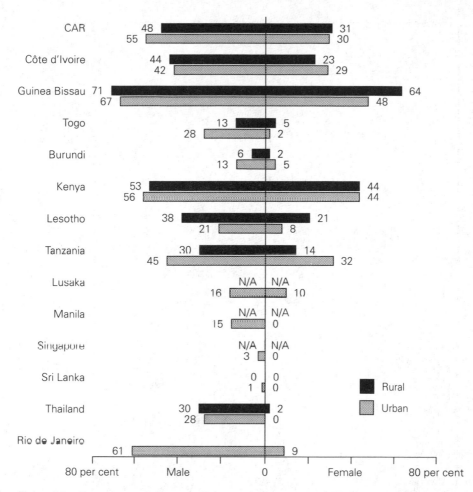

Figure 4.2:   Percentage of never-married men and women aged 15–19 years who reported sexual intercourse in the last 12 months, by residence (N/A: data not available)

cultural traditions are all factors that invalidate broad generalizations about urban–rural disparities. These factors also have different implications for the potential spread of HIV in rural areas. However, an important finding is the high correlation between the prevalence of premarital sexual activity in urban and rural settings as disclosed in Figure 4.3. The pattern shows that sexual behaviour among young people in cities and towns is closely related to sexual behaviour in rural areas.

Figure 4.4 shows the proportions of never-married males and females aged 15 to 19 who were sexually active among three educational levels that were standardized across countries: no education, primary education, secondary and higher education. Educational background has been shown to be a powerful predictor of many health-related behaviours (Cleland and van

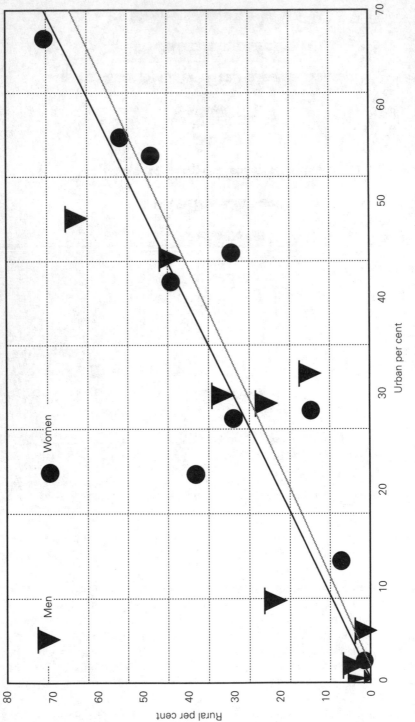

Figure 4.3: Relationship between percentages of urban and rural never-married men and women aged 15–19 years who reported sexual intercourse in the last 12 months

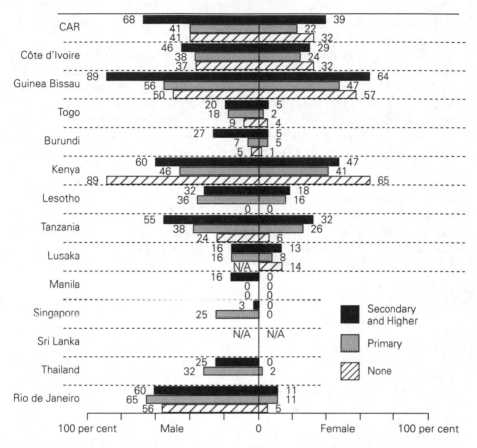

Figure 4.4: Percentage of never-married men and women aged 15–19 years who reported sexual intercourse in the last 12 months, by education level (N/A: data not available)

Ginneken, 1989). However, education is also well known to be confounded with other variables such as religion, ethnicity, age, urban residence, wealth and status. In presenting univariate analyses of the relationships between education and sexual behaviour, we should therefore refrain from inferring any direct causal link between the two factors.

For young men, sexual activity is more common among those with secondary schooling than among the primary and no schooling groups. There are only four exceptions (Kenya, Lesotho, Singapore and Thailand) to this generalization among the 12 study populations for which this comparison can be made. For women, the reported sexual behaviour of primary and secondary groups tends to be similar, but those with no schooling are less sexually active. There are three exceptions to this pattern (Côte d'Ivoire, Kenya and Lusaka), all among populations where premarital sex is generally common. This result suggests that education results in a relaxation of social controls on behaviour in societies where such controls are still forceful. In other societies, it makes little difference.

One further reason for the positive link between educational attainment and pre-nuptial sexual activity is that secondary schooling is incompatible with early marriage. In nearly all societies better educated men and women marry later than their less educated counterparts. To some extent, then, the education–premarital sex link merely reflects greater exposure to risk; the educated experience a longer span between puberty and first enduring partnership. Another possible explanation is opportunity. Attendance at secondary school may entail living away from parents in a town or a city, with a concomitant increase in freedom. Exposure to modern values of a sexually liberal nature is yet another possible cause. For young women, this appears to be a more likely explanation than opportunity because the main behavioural difference occurs between those with no schooling and those with primary or higher schooling. Attendance at primary school rarely implies living away from home but may inculcate new values.

Sexual Experience among 15–29 Year Olds

A more comprehensive approach to sexual initiation is gained by dropping the distinction between sex before and within marriage and analysing the proportion in each single year age group who have ever experienced intercourse. The data are presented in Figures 4.5. To smooth erratic fluctuations arising from the small number of respondents at each single year of age, a three-year moving average has been taken.

The huge cross-cultural variability in the onset of sexual behaviour is immediately apparent. In some societies, over half of 15 year olds are already sexually experienced. In other societies, nearly all are virgins at this age. At age 20, the level of sexual experience is close to 90 per cent in most of the study populations, but below 20 per cent in a minority. At the age of 29, virginity is very rare in most cases but is still over 40 per cent in a few instances.

Most of the African societies comprise a reasonably homogeneous group, with an early sexual debut and with no marked differences between males and females. At age 15, typically about 40 per cent of males and females have experienced intercourse, though this figure ranges from 35 to 60 per cent. At age 20, typically 80 per cent or more are experienced.

The two exceptions to this pattern are Burundi and Lesotho. At the age of 15, males in these two countries are just as likely to report sexual experience as males elsewhere in Africa. Thereafter, however, the upwards gradient is much more gentle than in other African surveys, and thus there is an increasing divergence. At age 20, for instance, about 40 per cent of men in Burundi and Lesotho report themselves to be virgins compared to a typical value of about 20 per cent in other African countries. This gap is still apparent

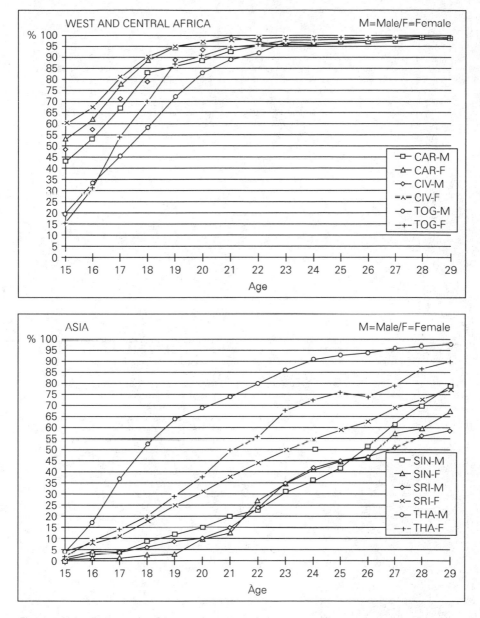

Figure 4.5(a):   Percentage of men and women who were sexually experienced, by current age (15–29 year olds)

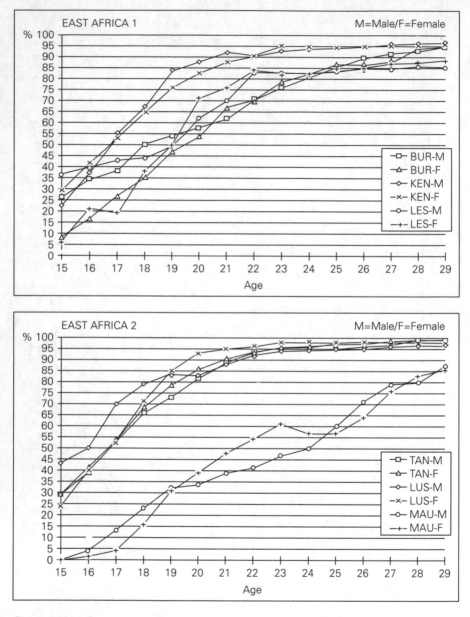

Figure 4.5(b): Percentage of men and women who were sexually experienced, by current age (15–29 year olds)

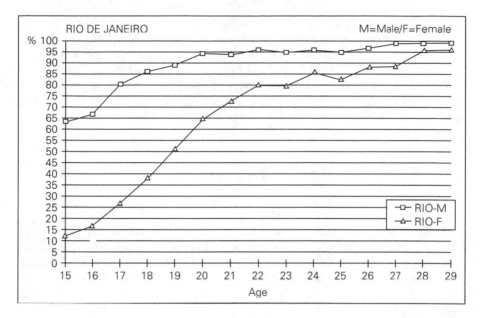

Figure 4.5(c): *Percentage of men and women who were sexually experienced, by current age (15–29 year olds)*

at age 29, though by then it has narrowed. For females the contrast takes a different form. At age 15, females in Burundi and Lesotho are much more likely to be virgins than elsewhere, and this difference is maintained at all higher ages.

Among the surveys conducted outside Africa, there are huge variations. Postponement of sexual initiation is most pronounced for Singaporean males and females. At age 20, over 80 per cent of both sexes report themselves to be virgins. At the age of 25, approximately 60 per cent are still inexperienced while, at age 29, the proportion has fallen only to about 40 per cent. Singapore is an extreme example of a late marrying population, with strong social controls on premarital sex for both men and women. The only other study population to match the Singapore results is males in Sri Lanka, another late marrying culture with an emphasis on virginity. In this country, females are much more likely to be sexually experienced at all ages from 15 to 29. The reason, of course, is not greater sexual laxity for women than men. It is simply a reflection that women marry at much younger ages than men.

In the two remaining populations, Rio de Janeiro and Thailand, men experience sex earlier than women. The disparity is particularly great in Rio de Janeiro. In this city, nearly 70 per cent of males aged 15 report sexual experience: a level higher than any recorded among the African surveys. The corresponding proportion for females in Rio de Janeiro is under 20 per cent. This gap narrows steadily and is very small by age 29. In Thailand, the male–female divergence is small at age 15; it widens at subsequent ages and then narrows after age 20. In both these societies, the main reason for the observed patterns is greater premarital intercourse for men than for women.

The median age at first sexual intercourse for males and females aged 15 to 29 – the age at which 50 per cent report having had sexual intercourse – further highlights regional differences (Figure 4.6). The contrast between sub-Saharan Africa and the Asian countries – including Mauritius – is clearly evident.

Virginity at First Regular Partnership

The analysis of premarital sex among young people does not allow a precise measure of the proportion of people who first experience intercourse with a regular partner or spouse. To estimate the proportion who enter marriage or stable partnership as virgins, we have calculated the number of people who reported identical ages for first intercourse and for first marriage. The assumption is made that the first sexual partner and the first spouse is the same in such cases. This analysis obviously has to be restricted to *ever-married* respondents and is further confined to those aged 25 to 49. By age 25, the majority of people in our study populations have married and therefore selection biases are minimized. There is, however, a disadvantage in concentrating attention on older respondents. Reliance has to be placed on the accurate recall of events that may have taken place many years ago. An internal consistency check reported in Chapter 2 showed that between 0 and 8 per cent of respondents reported a higher age at first sexual intercourse than age at first regular partnership; they were omitted in the following analysis. This level of inconsistency is low and suggests that the data are of reasonable quality.

In Figure 4.7, the results are summarized in terms of the proportions of persons whose first sexual intercourse was most probably with the first regular partner. The proportion of female virgins varies from 29 per cent in Kenya to 97 per cent in Thailand, showing that for a large majority of women – with the particular exception of Kenya – premarital chastity is still an important cultural value, especially for Asian women. Among men, the level of sexual experience before marriage is much higher than for women: virginity is reported by only 8 per cent in Kenya to a high of 64 per cent in Singapore, with a range for most of the surveys between 25 to 30 per cent.

In sub-Saharan Africa, female virginity before marriage is still the rule for a majority of women in three out of the four countries studied. According to Caldwell, Orubuloye and Caldwell (1992), the reason is perhaps not some abstract moral principle but the practical consideration that women should direct their sexuality into their most important social role, that of reproduction.

As shown in Table 4.3, the proportion of women classified as virgins at

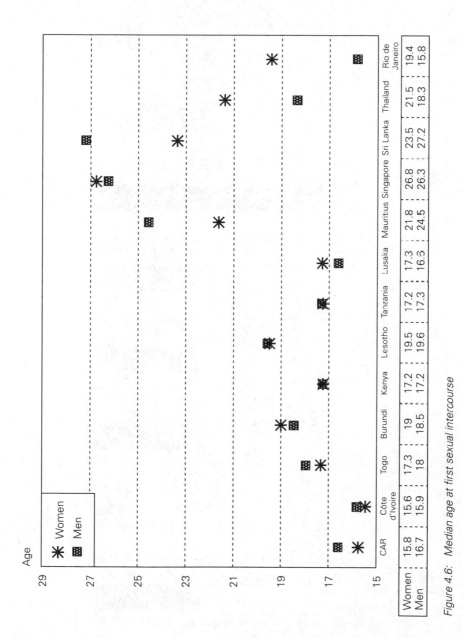

Figure 4.6: Median age at first sexual intercourse

	CAR	Côte d'Ivoire	Togo	Burundi	Kenya	Lesotho	Tanzania	Lusaka	Mauritius	Singapore	Sri Lanka	Thailand	Rio de Janeiro
Women	15.8	15.6	17.3	19	17.2	19.5	17.2	17.3	21.8	26.8	23.5	21.5	19.4
Men	16.7	15.9	18	18.5	17.2	19.6	17.3	16.5	24.5	26.3	27.2	18.3	15.8

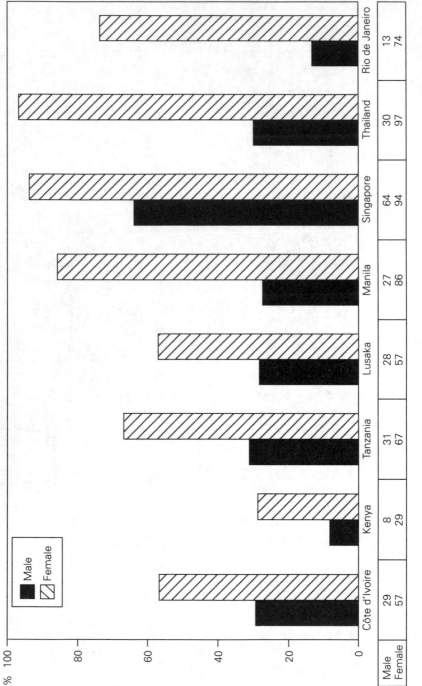

	Côte d'Ivoire	Kenya	Tanzania	Lusaka	Manila	Singapore	Thailand	Rio de Janeiro
Male	29	8	31	28	27	64	30	13
Female	57	29	67	57	86	94	97	74

Figure 4.7: Percentage who were virgins at time of first marriage/partnership, among ever-married men and women aged 25–49 years

Table 4.3: Percentage of ever-married men and women who were not sexually experienced at time of first marriage/partnership, by current age

	25–29	30–34	35–39	40–49
Côte d'Ivoire				
Male	35	24	23	29
Female	53	56	58	68
Kenya				
Male	15	8	5	6
Female	31	25	30	32
Tanzania				
Male	30	24	28	42
Female	66	77	82	83
Lusaka				
Male	38	26	23	28
Female	51	57	68	65
Manila				
Male	36	29	21	24
Female	83	88	85	87
Singapore				
Male	57	71	56	68
Female	92	95	95	94
Thailand				
Male	28	26	27	37
Female	98	96	95	99
Rio de Janeiro				
Male	17	14	9	13
Female	71	69	75	81

marriage is lower among younger than older age groups. However, one should also note evidence of a slight increase in reported virginity among 25 to 29-year-olds in Kenya, Thailand and Rio de Janeiro. This apparent reversal of the secular decline in premarital abstinence may be genuine: perhaps a reaction to the AIDS epidemic. Conversely, the finding may reflect greater accuracy of recall among younger women or the fact that not all women aged 25 to 29 have married.

At the societal level, female virginity at first marriage is related to female extra-marital sex in the last 12 months. Study populations with high levels of female virginity also reported low levels of female extra-marital sex among the 25–49 year olds ($R = 0.74$; $p = 0.03$). In other words, virginity is a good indicator of the strength of the societal control on female sexuality. Societies tend to unify rules on sexual behaviour around reproduction. The theory that low premarital sex might be associated with high extra-marital sex or vice versa, as suggested by modellers (Knolle, 1991) receives no support from the survey results. There were no statistical associations between female virginity and male virginity, or between female virginity and the reported occurrence of non-regular or commercial sex by men, or between male virginity and male extra-marital sex. Strict control on the sexual behaviour of women does not imply the existence of similar controls for men.

Duration of Sexual Exposure Before First Regular Partnership

The interval between first sexual intercourse and formation of first regular partnership, or marriage, is of particular interest for the HIV pandemic as an indicator of the length of potential exposure to HIV before the formation of a regular partnership. Clearly, entry into a marriage or regular partnership does not mean that risk behaviour will suddenly cease. Levels of divorce and separation may be high and extra-marital sex may occur. Nevertheless the length of time between first intercourse and first stable partnership remains a useful indicator of potential enhancement of risk: the longer the duration, the more likely it is that the number of sexual contacts will increase. Economic crises, declining incomes and housing difficulties have resulted in postponement of marriage in many societies though, to some extent, cohabitation and less formal relationships have replaced legal marriage (Caraël, 1993). There has also been concern about increases in premarital sexual intercourse in recent decades (United Nations, 1989).

The analysis was performed by computing, for each ever-married respondent, the difference between reported ages at first sex and at first marriage. As throughout this chapter, the term *marriage* is used broadly to denote any type of regular partnership. The focus of interest is again narrowed to respondents aged 25 to 49 years, and cautions concerning possible biases due to memory lapse should be repeated.

The mean duration is always longer for men than for women (Figure 4.8). Gender differences reflect the higher proportion of women than men having their first sexual intercourse around the time of first marriage. This is particularly noticeable among women in Asian populations, as already seen with the results on premarital chastity. Among men, intervals of more than five years are found in most countries, except in Asia. For men, reasons to delay marriage or cohabitation include bridewealth prices, pressures of poverty and difficulty of finding houses or land.

The amount of premarital exposure among younger and older male cohorts can be compared to detect changes over time. An historical trend towards increased premarital sexual behaviour has been documented by several authors (Feyisitan and Pebley, 1989; Konings, *et al.*, 1994). Delay in age at first marriage has also been reported by many authors as a result of increased female education and other factors (Lesthaeghe, 1989). These twin considerations lead us to expect that the length of premarital exposure will increase steadily from shorter durations among older cohorts to longer ones among younger people. However, the results in Figure 4.8 do not confirm this expectation. Indeed, among men in Manila and Rio de Janeiro, the opposite trend can be observed. In other surveys, there is a variety of patterns but

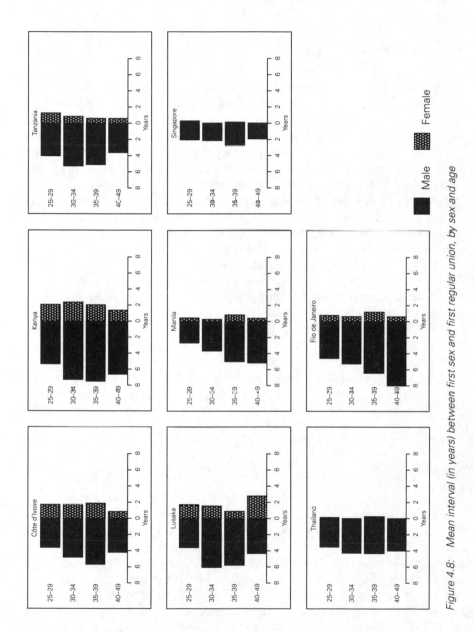

Figure 4.8:   Mean interval (in years) between first sex and first regular union, by sex and age

there is little clear-cut evidence of increasing exposure over time. The explanation may lie in an increase of informal partnerships that mitigate the effects of rising age at more formal marriage.

Sex Within Marriage

Throughout most developing countries a high value was traditionally placed on children, resulting in early and near-universal marriage and in buoyant fertility levels. Changes in nuptiality have been more rapid in cities than in rural areas, because an urban environment leads to greater social mobility, large income disparities, heterogenous populations and a partial breakdown of traditional controls over marriage and adolescent sexual life (Parkin and Nyamwaya, 1987; Nelson, 1988). In sub-Saharan Africa, new forms of sexual relationship have been flourishing in the last decade, especially in cities, explaining in part the higher urban rates of divorce and separation. In cities, married men tend to acquire sexual partners – some regular, others occasional – besides their spouse (Parkin and Nyamwaya, 1987). There is a continuum in such relationships from the concubine or the outside wife, to the *deuxième bureau* or *femme libre*, and to sex workers. In some urban areas of the third world, nearly half of the people are living in unions not legitimized by any formal agreement (Caraël, 1994).

The WHO/GPA surveys did not attempt to distinguish between these forms of relationships with their many subtle variations in obligations and expectations. The definition of marriage in these surveys was broad (see Chapter 2). It included all partnerships sanctified by law, religious ceremony or customary celebration but also included less formal unions, which two individuals regarded as forming a regular relationship, and any sexual union that had lasted for at least one year.

Current Marital Status

Marriage remains a central institution for the regulation of sexual behaviour. Marital status is known to affect the number of sexual partners and the frequency of sexual intercourse. Being in a formal marriage tends to reduce risk of HIV infection (e.g. Lindan, *et al.*, 1991). However, cultures vary in the nature and strength of the customs and sanctions controlling faithfulness in different types of unions. Moreover, the probability of early dissolution of first marriages and informal unions varies greatly. Answers to the question *Are you married or have a regular partner or are you widowed, divorced or separated?* allow us to describe current marital or partnership status.

Among male respondents aged 15 to 29 years, the proportion currently married (or with a regular partner) ranges from 19 to 64 per cent and, among females, from 25 to 81 per cent. In this age group, more females than males are currently in an enduring partnership. Gender differences in age at marriage and polygamy are responsible for this difference. Asian countries show a pattern of delayed marriage for both males and females consistent with lower levels of sexual activity. Not surprisingly, higher levels of separation occur among the youngest age groups when informal unions are more common. The prevalence of separation, divorce, and widowhood varies from 0 to 10 per cent across countries, with the lowest proportion in Singapore and the highest among men in Guinea Bissau (10 per cent) and women in the Central African Republic, Guinea Bissau, Lesotho and Lusaka (5 per cent). Widowhood is very uncommon among persons aged 15 to 29 years.

Median Age at First Marriage

Figure 4.9 shows the median age at first marriage, or regular partnership, using current status data to identify the age at which 50 per cent is married. Among men, the median ranges from 19 to 28 years and, among women, from 17 to 27 years. The median is always younger for women than for men, with a difference ranging from 1 year in Singapore to 5 years in Kenya, Mauritius and Tanzania. In continental sub-Saharan Africa, the age at marriage for women is not universally young. The median value for the eight populations surveyed varies from 17 to 20 years. Age at marriage tends to be later in east and southern Africa than in west and central Africa. The timing of first marriage in the Asian study populations is typically later than in Africa for both men and women.

For the last 20 years, ages at marriage in many countries have risen in response to socio-economic development and rises in female education (United Nations, 1987). Between women with no education and those with seven or more years of schooling, the difference in age at marriage ranges from three to seven years. Even modest exposure to primary education produces a delayed entry into regular sexual partnerships for women. This effect is found in both rural and urban areas but is more apparent in the latter where educational opportunities for women are better.

Age Difference between Spouses/Regular Partners

An important factor in explaining variations in levels of HIV infection is the age difference between sexual partners. As premarital sexual activity usually increases among persons who marry late, a large gap between the ages of spouses may mean that women are at increased risk of HIV infection via their male partner. In WHO/GPA surveys, the mean age gap between spouses at first marriage ranges from 3 to 10 years. In Rio de Janeiro, Thailand, Sri

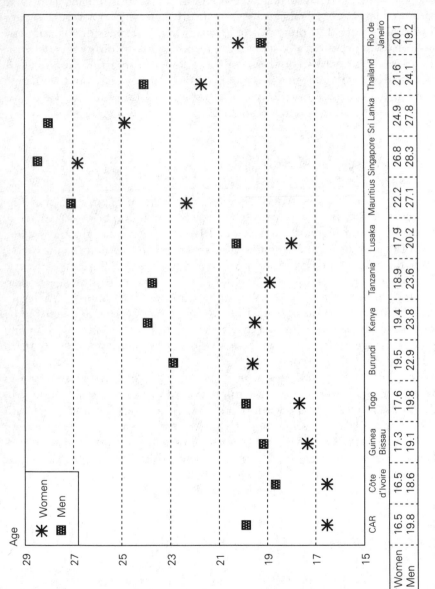

Figure 4.9: Median age at first marriage/partnership

	CAR	Côte d'Ivoire	Guinea Bissau	Togo	Burundi	Kenya	Tanzania	Lusaka	Mauritius	Singapore	Sri Lanka	Thailand	Rio de Janeiro
Women	16.5	16.5	17.3	17.6	19.5	19.4	18.9	17.9	22.2	26.8	24.9	21.6	20.1
Men	19.8	18.6	19.1	19.8	22.9	23.8	23.6	20.2	27.1	28.3	27.8	24.1	19.2

Lanka and Singapore, the average age difference is about 3 to 4 years and there is a good agreement between spouses on their mutual ages.

In Tanzania and Côte d'Ivoire, where polygynous marriages are common, women reported that their partners, on average, are older than themselves by 9 to 10 years. Men, however, reported a smaller average gap of 6 to 7 years. The question asked to male respondent was, *How old is your wife/ regular partner?* with the instruction: *If the respondent says he/she has more than one spouse/partner, ask about the main partner.* High levels of polygyny appear to be associated with early female age at first partnership and large age differences between spouses. In these two countries, there was a continuous increase in the age difference between spouses with ascending male ages: in Côte d'Ivoire, a 4-year difference is observed in the group aged 20 to 24 as compared to a 12.4-year difference in the group aged 40 to 49; in Tanzania, the corresponding differences are 3 years and 9.6 years.

Polygyny and Multiple Partnerships

Among the different types of relationship, the more stable ones – when they are mutually monogamous and neither partner is infected – carry less HIV risk than more transitory ones. However, polygyny may influence sexual behaviour in many ways that are relevant for HIV infection. Respondents were asked, *Do you now have one or more than one spouse/regular partner; IF MORE THAN ONE, how many?* WHO/GPA surveys do not permit us to distinguish formal polygamous marriage from multiple regular partnerships that carry less social recognition.

There is a wide variation in the prevalence of multiple current partnerships; among men aged 15 to 49 years, the range is from 0.2 per cent to 55 per cent (Figure 4.10 left side). Low values of around 2 to 3 per cent are typical of men in Asian countries, with even fewer women reporting multiple partners. Among the African study sites, Lesotho has the highest level, for men and for women, although formalized polygyny is low by African standards. A survey in 1977 found that only 9 per cent of married women were living in polygynous unions. The very high labour migration, affecting more than half of the adult male population, appears to have resulted in the weakening of marriage and a rise of open concubinage (Murray, 1977).

Men in Côte d'Ivoire, Kenya, Lusaka and Tanzania also reported high levels of multiple partnership. One can only speculate that, perhaps at early ages, many women are concubines and at older ages most of them are polygynous spouses. As mentioned earlier, WHO/GPA surveys do not permit us to distinguish between these differing types of relationship. According to Wa Karanja (1987), an *outside* wife involves separate residence, a duration of several years, financial support of the woman by the man, the legitimation of the children and the acceptance of a low social status by the woman. But, again according to Wa Karanja, the status of outside wives is not necessarily

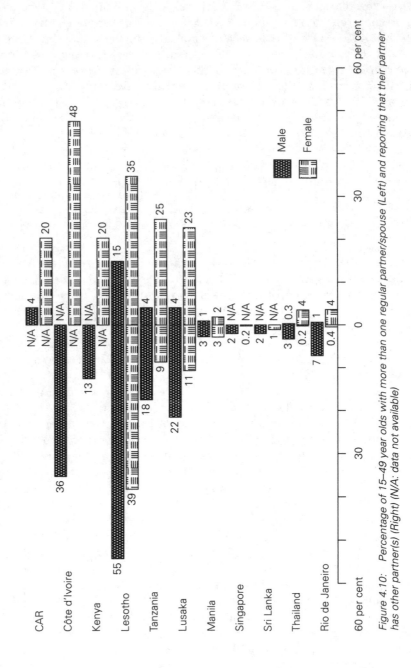

Figure 4.10: Percentage of 15–49 year olds with more than one regular partner/spouse (Left) and reporting that their partner has other partner(s) (Right) (N/A: data not available)

perceived as less satisfactory than the status of fully recognized wives by the women themselves because the former situation confers greater independence.

The proportion of women in Tanzania and Lusaka who reported more than one regular partner is around 10 per cent, suggesting that a minority of women is relying on more than one partner for their support. Not surprisingly, in Lesotho, this proportion is as high as 39 per cent, with a few variations by age. This pattern again reflects the temporary migration of more than half of the adult male population to the Republic of South Africa that leaves couples separated for most of the year. In Singapore, Thailand and Manila, less than one per cent of women reported more than one regular partner.

Risk of HIV infection depends not only on personal risk behaviour but on the behaviour of the spouse or regular partner. A further question was asked to respondents currently in union whether they think that their partner has other partners than themselves. The question did not relate specifically to regular partner but the context was within a discussion of regular relationships.

As shown in Figure 4.10 (right side), there is a striking difference between answers of men and women. With the exception of Lesotho – where 15 per cent reported that their wife had other partners – the proportions of men who thought that their female partner had other partners were very low, ranging from 0.3 to 4.8 per cent. For women, the corresponding proportion was nearly 50 per cent in Côte d'Ivoire and Togo, and between 15 and 25 per cent in the other African surveys. In the Asian sites again, the picture was very different; the proportion was only around 3 per cent.

When comparing the eight surveys for which we have data, there is a strong relationship between the proportion of men reporting more than one partner and the proportion of women reporting that their husbands have multiple partners. The correlation was highly significant (R = 0.85; p = 0.002). If Lesotho is considered as an outlier and removed, the correlation coefficient rises to 0.98.

It is expected that age at marriage for women will be inversely correlated with the level of multiple partnerships among men. In other words, high proportions of men with more than one regular partner will be associated with lower median age at marriage for women. This is indeed the case for the eight surveys for which such data are available (R = 0.84; p = 0.01).

There was also a significant positive correlation between the proportion of men with more than one regular partner and the proportion of married men reporting sex outside of regular partnerships in the last 12 months (R = 0.85; p = 0.002). This link, shown in Figure 4.11, suggests that polygamous values influence the prevalence of extra-marital relations as well, though it is dangerous to generalize from such a small sample of societies. Finally, we may note that there was no association between the proportion of males reporting more than one regular partner and the prevalence of male or female premarital sex.

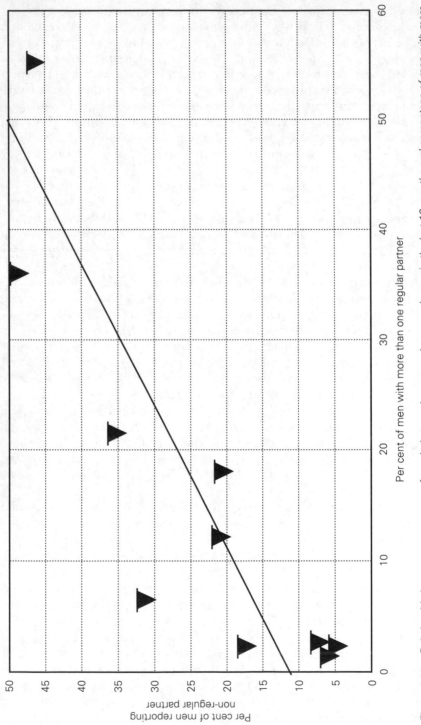

Per cent of men with more than one regular partner

Per cent of men reporting
non-regular partner

Figure 4.11: Relationship between percentage of married men who reported non-regular sex in the last 12 months and percentage of men with more than one spouse/regular partner

Table 4.4: *Percentage of married men and women who were not cohabiting with principal spouse/partner, by age*

	Males					Females				
	Age					Age				
	25–29	30–34	35–39	40–49	All 15–49	25–29	30–34	35–39	40–49	All 15–49
Côte d'Ivoire	47	19	8	8	43	26	19	21	16	36
Kenya	26	17	18	21	20	20	23	17	21	20
Lesotho	29	34	30	27	31	25	23	28	30	24
Tanzania	14	7	7	4	11	15	16	11	9	15
Lusaka	35	23	5	5	31	18	12	10	10	26
Manila	5	7	9	0	6	13	10	5	2	8
Singapore	29	8	3	5	12	5	2	2	2	4
Sri Lanka	7	5	4	5	5	3	6	8	5	6
Thailand	3	5	2	6	4	16	12	11	10	13
Rio de Janeiro	34	22	15	9	25	36	12	19	12	24

Non-cohabiting Partnerships

A measure of cohabitation in WHO/GPA questionnaires was obtained through the very simple question, *Do you and your wife/regular partner live together in the same household?* The question was obviously restricted to married respondents. For respondents with more than one current partner, the question was restricted to the main partner, that is, the person seen most frequently. The results in Table 4.4 demonstrate the importance of non-cohabitation, owing perhaps to seasonal or permanent migration, especially among young males. Non-cohabitation is most common at ages 25 to 34. In African surveys, large proportions of currently married respondents – between 11 and 43 per cent – reported that they are not cohabiting.

In the Asian study populations, non-cohabiting partnerships are much less common, but in Rio de Janeiro, the level is similar to those found in Africa. In countries with high levels of polygyny or multiple regular relationships, one should not expect the extent of cohabitation to be equal between men and women. In polygynous marriages, non-cohabitation is often the rule: men rotate from one spouse to the other. This pattern implies that more women than men should report non-cohabitation; this is the case to a certain extent in Tanzania but not elsewhere in Africa.

Where married men migrate away from home and find a new female partner, they might report non-cohabitation in reference to their primary marriage; under these circumstances, more men than women would report non-cohabitation, as occurs in Côte d'Ivoire, Lesotho, Lusaka and in Singapore. Another possible explanation is that men and women attach different meanings to the concept of living together; a woman may be more likely than a man to report that her partner is living with her, even if co-residence is sporadic.

As expected, at the aggregate level, there is a significant association between the level of male non-cohabitation and the proportion of men reporting more than one regular partner. The correlation is significant for the ten surveys where data have been collected (R = 0.74; p = 0.01). As suggested by Capron and Kohler (1975), polygyny and male emigration are mutually reinforcing. The absence of young men gives older, wealthier men, who remain at home, more opportunities for monopolizing the pool of available women.

There is a close association between the proportion of males in non-cohabiting partnerships and the frequency of non-regular sex within the last 12 months. For 10 surveys, Figure 4.12 displays the relationship between the proportion of married men and women who report sexual contacts outside of marriage and the proportion of married men and women reporting non-cohabitation (R = 0.92; p = 0.0002 for men, and R = 0.76; p = 0.01 for women). This finding is important in revealing how the nature of the marital bond is expressed, though cohabitation may influence sexual behaviour outside of marriage.

Sexual Activity and Coital Frequency with Spouse

Respondents in regular partnerships were asked whether they had sexual intercourse with (any) regular partner during the last 12 months and during the last month. They were also asked about frequency of intercourse with their partner in the last four weeks. Table 4.5 shows the distributions of males and females according to reported marital sex. The proportions reporting abstinence in the last 12 months range from 0 to 12 per cent with the single exception of women in Togo (24 per cent). Women were more likely than men to report no sexual intercourse within the last 12 months, especially in Togo, Manila and Côte d'Ivoire. Lactational taboos and polygyny may account for these differences. The same types of explanation may apply to the proportions sexually inactive within the last month. Unexpectedly large proportions of men and women reported no sex during the last month, more so in Africa than elsewhere. Among the African respondents, between 32 and 59 per cent report no sex with a regular partner in the last month. Among the non-African populations surveyed, abstinence from intercourse is moderate in Sri Lanka and Manila (about 30 per cent), less common in Singapore and lower still in Thailand and Rio de Janeiro.

The reference period for the number of sexual acts between spouses in WHO/GPA surveys was four weeks. Other studies have shown that respondents attempt to estimate their coital frequency in terms of either a typical week or the past week, and multiply this number by the number of weeks in the reference period (Westoff, 1974; Blanc and Rutenberg, 1991). Respondents may also provide normative responses that reflect what they perceive to be a socially acceptable level. Interpretative caution is therefore necessary.

The relevant questions were restricted to married respondents who reported previously that they were sexually active with their spouse in the last month. In WHO/GPA surveys, the question asked was, *In the last 4 weeks, that*

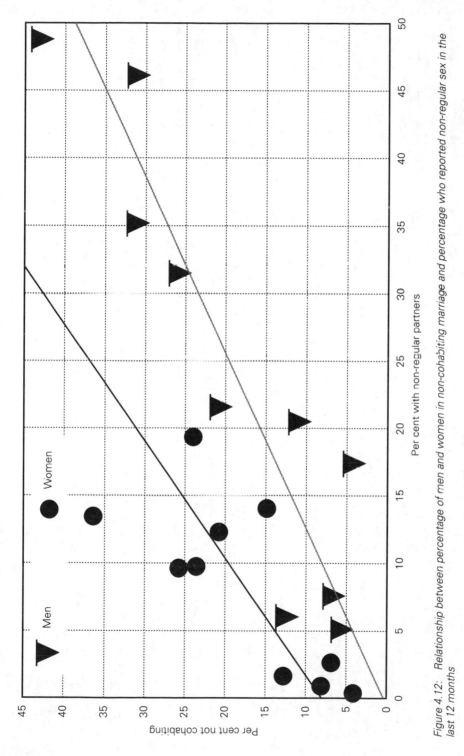

Figure 4.12: Relationship between percentage of men and women in non-cohabiting marriage and percentage who reported non-regular sex in the last 12 months

Table 4.5: Percentage of currently married respondents aged 15-49 years who have had sexual intercourse with their regular partner during the last 12 months and during the last month, and mean coital frequency during the last month

	Côte d'Ivoire		Togo		Burundi		Lesotho		Tanzania		Lusaka	
	M	F	M	F	M	F	M	F	M	F	M	F
Per cent no sex this year	4	8	11	24	6	8	4	6	6	8	2	2
Per cent sex this year but no sex this month	38	42	31	34	27	26	46	54	28	28	42	43
Per cent sex this month	58	50	58	42	68	66	50	41	66	64	56	55
Mean coital frequency												
Age 15–19	2.2	1.8	1.9	1.1	1.9	4.5	1.2	1.0	4.6	5.4	1.0	2.6
20–24	2.5	2.2	1.9	1.5	4.9	7.0	1.6	1.7	4.2	4.1	2.1	3.9
25–29	3.0	1.9	2.9	1.9	6.2	6.3	3.6	2.1	5.1	4.6	3.9	4.7
30–34	3.0	2.1	3.8	1.4	5.5	6.2	3.6	2.2	5.3	4.6	4.4	4.0
35–39	2.8	2.0	2.7	1.5	6.2	5.4	2.8	2.2	4.7	4.5	4.3	4.1
40–49	3.2	1.5	3.6	1.5	5.7	4.0	3.8	2.1	5.0	3.6	3.0	1.8
All 15–49	2.9	2.0	2.9	1.5	5.5	5.7	3.0	1.9	4.9	4.4	3.4	3.7
N	865	1136	811	961	735	826	356	805	1119	1642	594	738

	Manila		Singapore		Sri Lanka		Thailand		Rio de Janeiro	
	M	F	M	F	M	F	M	F	M	F
Per cent no sex this year	7	12	0	0	5	7	1	2	0	1
Per cent sex this year but no sex this month	22	21	13	13	29	22	11	14	6	6
Per cent sex this month	71	67	87	87	66	71	89	84	94	93
Mean coital frequency										
Age 15–19	3.6	1.0	0.3	1.7	1.8	4.1	6.3	7.5	10.2	6.1
20–24	2.8	3.1	1.6	3.3	3.9	5.7	6.9	5.4	8.9	8.3
25–29	3.1	3.3	3.6	4.6	5.3	6.0	6.7	5.5	9.4	8.2
30–34	3.6	3.0	4.5	3.9	4.1	4.3	6.1	4.5	9.0	8.9
35–39	3.4	2.8	3.9	3.3	5.0	3.8	5.8	4.1	8.3	8.0
40–49	2.7	2.1	3.4	2.8	3.3	2.7	4.2	2.6	7.9	5.6
All 15–49	2.9	2.5	3.6	3.4	4.1	4.1	5.7	4.3	8.7	7.6
N	282	418	505	606	843	900	703	1133	415	487

is since last . . . , have you had sex with your spouse/regular partner? IF YES, how many times in the last 4 weeks?

There are many potential determinants of coital frequency: co-residence; the prevalence of polygyny; the extent of customary restrictions on intercourse, for example, during pregnancy or in the post-partum period; sex-specific migration patterns or seasonal burden of work and non-regular sex. This analysis, however, is restricted to an initial descriptive presentation of results and no attempt is made to examine the determinants of coital frequency, as, for instance, in Faulkenberry, *et al.* (1987) and Blanc and Rutenberg (1991).

The mean coital frequency (among all married respondents, sexually active or not) in the four weeks prior to the interview ranges from a maximum of 8.7 sexual acts in Rio de Janeiro to a minimum of 1.5 in Togo. The striking feature of the results is the generally low frequency of intercourse. In about half of the study populations, the overall mean is less than 4.0. In most sites, males report a higher frequency than females; the difference is particularly marked in Côte d'Ivoire, Togo and Lesotho, perhaps a reflection of polygyny. Nevertheless, there was a close correlation between male and female coital frequency at the aggregate level (R = 0.94; p = 0.0001).

The large differences between these study populations are consistent with the findings of other studies. The figures for Rio de Janeiro and Burundi were similar to those reported in other surveys for married women (Blanc and Rutenberg, 1991). Few studies have been able to provide explanations for differentials. The only clear pattern that emerges from the literature is declining coital frequency with increasing age and marital duration. That was confirmed in most populations surveyed by WHO/GPA with a peak in coital frequency among 25–34 year olds, and a decrease thereafter.

Non-regular and Commercial Sex

Measurement of the prevalence of high risk behaviours over time is needed to monitor changes in specific populations and to evaluate health education campaigns and other interventions. Initial assessment of various risk groups or risk behaviours is essential in determining intervention priorities. Moreover, an understanding of the predictors, or correlates, of risky sexual behaviours is useful to design or modify intervention programmes. Assessment in the area of sexual behaviour has been weakened considerably because there was no existing body of quantitative data on pre- and extra-marital sex. Moreover, the few studies that have been conducted differ in the variables measured, the reference periods and the population groups studied. Many of the samples are unrepresentative.

The WHO/GPA surveys attempted to make progress by providing researchers with standardized procedures, interview schedules and concepts. Key methodological precautions such as confidentiality, pre-tests of instruments, training of interviewers, and the matching of respondent and interviewer for age and gender were proposed as means to improve validity. At the same time, it was stressed that, because of the highly private nature of sexual behaviour, total reliance should not be placed on data elicited in face-to-face structured interviews. Results of specific tests of reliability and validity, sponsored by WHO/GPA are not yet available. In their absence, the results that follow should be interpreted with caution.

In WHO/GPA surveys, casual or non-regular sex means sex with a person who is not a spouse or regular partner (see earlier definition of regular partner). Among those reporting non-regular partners, a further question separates commercial and non-commercial casual relationships. *In the last 12 months, have you ever given or received any money, gifts or favour in return for sex?* The instructions to the interviewers emphasize that money, gifts or favours may be exchanged between two partners but that, if the exchange was not the prime motive or reason for sex, the relationship was not one of commercial sex. However, as discussed in Chapter 2, the distinction could have had different meanings in different cultures, which complicates intercountry comparisons. Little (1973) had proposed as a definition of a prostitute in the African context 'a person whose means of subsistence over a period of time depends wholly on the sale of sexual services and whose relationship with a customer does not extend beyond the sexual act.' This definition of the prostitute–client relationship is not entirely satisfactory and covers only one limited aspect of an often complex, ongoing relationship, although an important component is always the financial aspect.

The definition adopted for commercial sex in the WHO/GPA surveys was certainly a broad one and should not be considered equivalent to prostitution in the Western sense. The results on commercial sex that follow suffer from a lack of clarity of the underlying concepts but they reflect nonetheless an important aspect of the epidemiology of STD/HIV. All the figures and tables in this section use as their denominator the general population aged 15–49, including virgins, respondents who have had no sexual intercourse during the reference period, and those who have had intercourse exclusively with their regular partner. Figure 4.13 presents, for each survey, the proportion of male and female respondents 15 to 49 years old who reported non-regular but not commercial sex and those who reported commercial sex in the last 12 months. It should be noted that those who reported commercial sex may also have experienced non-commercial sex outside stable partnerships.

Sex Outside Regular Partnerships

Among males, the prevalence of sex outside of regular partnerships in the last 12 months ranges from 2 to 51 per cent, with a median of 28 per cent. Among females, the corresponding values are from 1 per cent to 19 per cent,

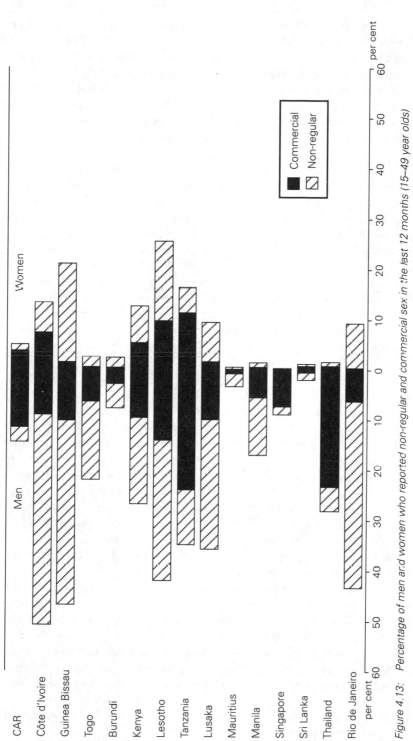

Figure 4.13: Percentage of men and women who reported non-regular and commercial sex in the last 12 months (15–49 year olds)

with a median of 8 per cent. Results from Burundi where the prevalence of seropositivity for HIV in 1990, among urban adults, was 19.2 per cent among females and 10.2 per cent among men are surprisingly low (PNLS, 1991).

The male–female ratio of non-regular sex was between two and three (twice to three times as many men than women) in sub-Saharan Africa with the exception of Côte d'Ivoire, Lusaka and Togo where it was even higher. In Asian countries, where the exchange of money for sexual acts, close to the restricted concept of prostitution, is an important part of sex outside marriage, the ratio of non-regular sex is systematically higher: 10 to 20 times more men than women report this type of sexual relationship. The reliance of men on female sex workers is certainly the major factor in the explanation of differences between gender, especially in Asian countries. Sex workers were probably not represented in any numbers in WHO/GPA surveys. Women are also more expected to be faithful to their regular partner and this social constraint may have led to considerable underreporting. At the population level, one would expect an association between reported non-regular sex among men and women. Indeed, the correlation of female and male non-regular sex is highly significant (R = 0.79; p = 0.001).

The proportion reporting at least one sex partner outside marriage in the last 12 months varied considerably by current marital status for both men and women. The formerly married usually had the highest proportion, followed by the never-married and the currently married (with the exception of Togo where the currently married are more likely to report such contacts). Table 4.6 takes the example of Côte d'Ivoire to show the per cent distribution of all respondents according to number of sexual associates apart from spouse/regular partner, if any, by current age and background characteristics. Formerly and never-married persons report nearly the same prevalence of risk behaviour. The prevalence of non-regular sex (including commercial sex) and the number of these temporary partners in the last 12 months was usually highest among 20 to 29 year olds men and among women aged 15 to 24 years. Single men aged 25 to 29 were more likely to report casual sex than the other groups. In most surveys, there was a higher reported level of sex outside marriage for both men and women in urban settings than in rural ones, with the exception of females in Thailand and Togo, but the levels in these two sites were very low (Figure 4.14).

In many societies, urbanization increases opportunities for sexual encounters and provides new models for sexual behaviour. The results suggest that urbanization and modernization favour transgression of the more restrictive traditions that exist in some rural areas. As more people marry late and as more relationships become informal, higher risk behaviours tend to concentrate in cities and towns. However, this difference does not mean that the extent of casual sex in rural and urban areas is not correlated. On the contrary, the more non-regular sex in rural areas for both men and women, the more there is in urban areas, as is shown in Figure 4.15 (for males R = 0.96, p = 0.0001; for females R = 0.91, p = 0.0002).

Table 4.6(a): Per cent distribution of all male and female respondents in the Côte d'Ivoire survey according to number of sexual associates (apart from spouse/partner, if any) in the last 12 months, by current age

Current Age	Sex	0	1	2–4	5+	Total
15–19	M	53	18	20	9	100
	F	81	10	9	0	100
20–24	M	38	14	34	13	100
	F	83	9	7	1	100
25–29	M	37	16	32	14	100
	F	91	4	5	0	100
30–34	M	52	15	24	9	100
	F	88	6	5	1	100
35–39	M	64	11	22	3	100
	F	95	3	3	0	100
40–49	M	70	13	15	1	100
	F	93	4	3	0	100
50+	M	80	7	10	3	100
	F	98	1	2	0	100
All 15–49	M	49	15	26	10	100
	F	87	7	6	1	100
All	M	54	14	24	9	100
	F	88	6	6	1	100

Table 4.6(b): Percentage of male and female respondents in the Côte d'Ivoire survey who reported at least one sexual associate (apart from current spouse/partner, if any) in the last 12 months, by current marital status and by residence and education

Background Characteristic	Sex	Currently	Formerly	Never	All
Residence					
Urban	M	48	61	55	51
	F	11	32	32	16
Rural	M	39	48	52	41
	F	7	24	19	9
Education					
No School	M	24	44	45	29
	F	6	25	29	9
Primary	M	38	53	50	42
	F	11	32	25	14
Secondary and High	M	60	68	60	60
	F	16	40	33	20
All 15–49	M	49	61	54	51
	F	10	38	29	13
All	M	43	55	54	46
	F	9	29	29	13

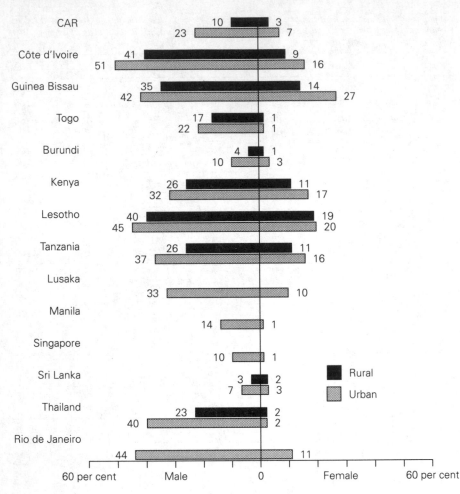

Figure 4.14: Percentage of all men and women who reported non-regular sex in the last 12 months, by residence

The male and female prevalence of non-regular sex in the last 12 months varies according to the three levels of education that were categorized in the surveys: no schooling, primary education, secondary and more (Figure 4.16). In most study populations there was a trend towards a higher prevalence among respondents with higher educational level. However, as for premarital sex, the effect of education was more evident for women at the level of primary and secondary education versus no schooling. For men, the effect was more apparent with the passage from primary to secondary and higher educational level. Logistic regression confirmed that the effect of education on casual sex was independent from the other variables.

There was a significant relationship between the prevalence of premarital sex among youths and the level of sex outside marriage among men

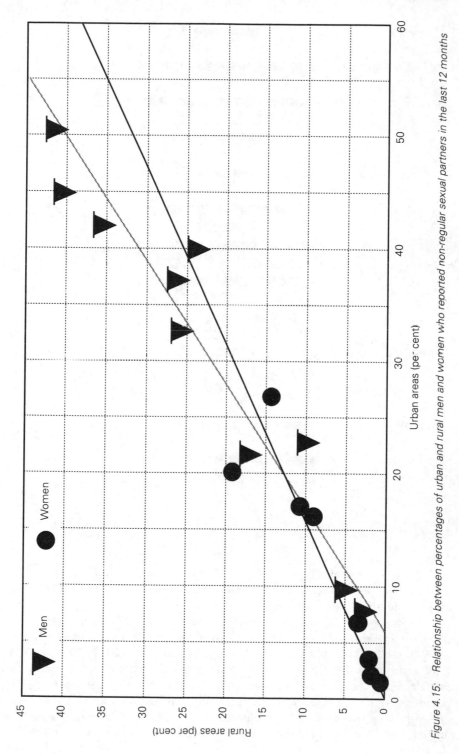

Figure 4.15: Relationship between percentages of urban and rural men and women who reported non-regular sexual partners in the last 12 months

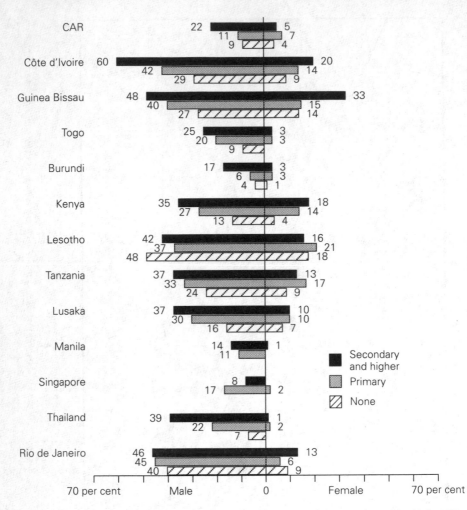

Figure 4.16: Percentage of all men and women who reported non-regular sex in the last 12 months, by education level

and women (for males R = 0.66, p = 0.007; for females R = 0.76, p = 0.002). This link highlights the existence of different consistent patterns of sexuality and a continuity from adolescence to adult ages.

People with a high rate of change of sexual partners have been shown to play a disproportionate role in the spread of sexually transmitted diseases, including HIV (Winkelstein, *et al.*, 1987; Anderson, *et al.*, 1991). For respondents reporting at least one sexual partner other than the regular one in the last 12 months, a question was asked about the number of such non-regular partners. Figure 4.17 illustrates the proportion of male and female respondents reporting five or more casual partners in the last 12 months, among 15–49 year olds. Among the 14 surveys, the proportions for men varied from 11

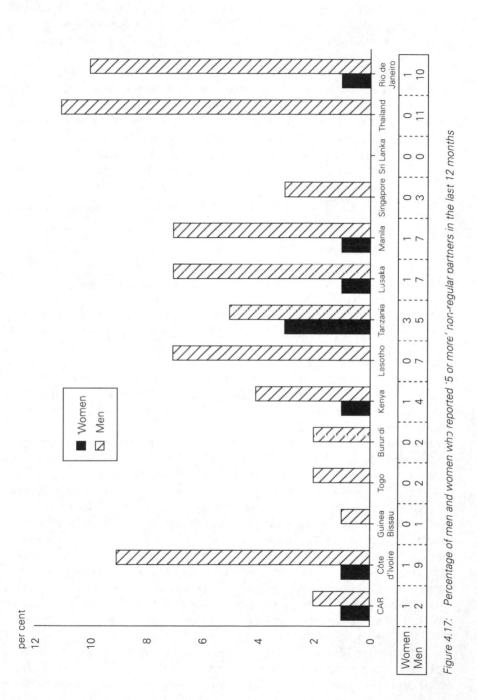

	CAR	Côte d'Ivoire	Guinea Bissau	Togo	Burundi	Kenya	Lesotho	Tanzania	Lusaka	Manila	Singapore	Sri Lanka	Thailand	Rio de Janeiro
Women	1	1	0	0	0	1	0	3	1	1	0	0	0	1
Men	2	9	1	2	2	4	7	5	7	7	3	0	11	10

Figure 4.17: Percentage of men and women who reported '5 or more' non-regular partners in the last 12 months

per cent in Thailand to 0 per cent in Sri Lanka; levels for women varied little, from 0 per cent in seven surveys to 3 per cent in Tanzania. The proportion of male respondents with more than five non-regular partners was consistently highest among the middle age range of 25 to 39 years.

For 13 surveys where data were available, there was a significant correlation between the aggregate prevalence among men of non-regular sex in the last 12 months and the per centage of male respondents with more than 5 casual partners ($R = 0.87$; $p = 0.0003$). In other words, one can expect higher heterogeneity and larger core groups of high transmitters when the general level of extra-marital sex is already high. Surprisingly, there was no correlation between the proportion of male respondents with 5 or more non-regular partners and the reported level of commercial sex by men, nor with the proportion of women reporting casual sex.

Commercial Sex

The proportion of all adults aged 15–49 reporting contacts with sex workers (at least one sexual encounter in the last 12 months where money or gifts were exchanged) among men ranged from 1 per cent in Sri Lanka to 24.7 per cent in Tanzania, with a median of 9.7 per cent and, among women, from 0.1 per cent in many countries to 11.2 per cent in Tanzania, with a median of 1.3 per cent (see Figure 4.13). The rather broad definition adopted in WHO/GPA surveys may have been interpreted differently by men and women. In Tanzania, its local meaning was particulay general and it is likely that many men and women who were not clients of sex workers or workers themselves, responded affirmatively to this item. Furthermore, it is likely that women substantially involved in sex work will not be adequately represented in a household survey and/or that the few women who reported commercial sex had many male clients. The WHO/GPA surveys do not permit a numerical breakdown of all recent non-marital partners into those of a commercial nature and others. Nevertheless, the number of men who reported commercial sex in the last 12 months in relation to the total number reporting non-marital sex of any kind provides a reasonable indication of the contribution of commercial sex to all non-marital encounters. In Rio de Janeiro and Côte d'Ivoire, men who reported commercial sex comprise 20 per cent or less of all those who reported any non-regular sexual contact. In most of the other study populations, the proportions vary between 25 and 40 per cent but are much higher (75 per cent or more) in the Central African Republic, Tanzania, Thailand and Singapore.

Unattached men – soldiers, travellers, traders, students, migrants – probably desire access to unattached women. Such relationships are not always associated with the negative stereotypes common in Europe and North America. In Rio de Janeiro and Côte d'Ivoire where the prevalence of non-regular sex among men was respectively 23 and 42 per cent, the relative importance of commercial sex is lower as compared to the other sexual interactions.

In all populations, contact with sex workers is more prevalent in urban than in rural areas. In all sites, except Lesotho, levels are also higher among formerly and never-married than among those with a regular partner. In the Asian study populations, commercial sex is almost entirely concentrated among single men. There is no marked age pattern to the reporting of commercial sex, though, as for casual sex, the proportion reporting commercial sex is usually the highest among men aged 20 to 29. There was a significant but weak correlation between the proportions of women reporting commercial sex and casual sex (R = 0.66; p = 0.01) but no correlation among men.

Of particular importance for the prevention of the spread of HIV is the use of condoms during sex in exchange of money or gifts. WHO/GPA surveys inquired about this issue by asking a single question to respondents who reported commercial sex in the last year; *Did you ever use a condom on these occasions? IF YES, Was it each time or sometimes?* Figure 4.18 discloses the per cent distribution of men according to condom use in commercial sex. The proportion of men who never used a condom varied from around 80 per cent in Togo, Tanzania, Manila and Rio de Janeiro to 25 per cent in Singapore. In Lusaka and Burundi, two areas where the HIV epidemic and the awareness of AIDS are high, more than 50 per cent of the men report condom use sometimes or always. In the Central African Republic, Côte d'Ivoire, Kenya, Lesotho and Tanzania where appreciable numbers of women (more than 30) reported commercial sex, the proportion never using condoms was consistently higher than for men, around 70 to 80 per cent. The implication is that women who are involved in commercial sex were less aware of sexually transmitted diseases and HIV than men. Further analysis of knowledge, ever-use and attitudes towards condoms may be found in Chapter 5.

Thus far, determinants of sexual behaviour have been explored by bivariate analyses. In an attempt to elucidate further the strength of independent and interactive effects, logistic regression was performed. A set of socio-demographic variables was selected from the preliminary analyses: these were current age, level of schooling, current marital status and urban-rural residence. In addition, drinking habits (drinking alcohol at least once a week – see Chapter 7) and perceived personal risk of HIV infection (see Chapter 6) were also included. Literacy, province, ethnicity, religion and selected psychological variables such as perceived threat of AIDS, locus of control, perceived severity of AIDS disease were excluded from the logistic regressions after exploratory analysis.

Separate regressions were conducted for men and women on a sub-set of six surveys on the binary variable *risk behaviour*. This outcome variable distinguished respondents who had one or more non-regular sexual partners in the last 12 months, including commercial sex, from respondents reporting no such sexual contacts. Condom use in commercial sex, although clearly affecting risk of STD infection, was not taken into account because reported

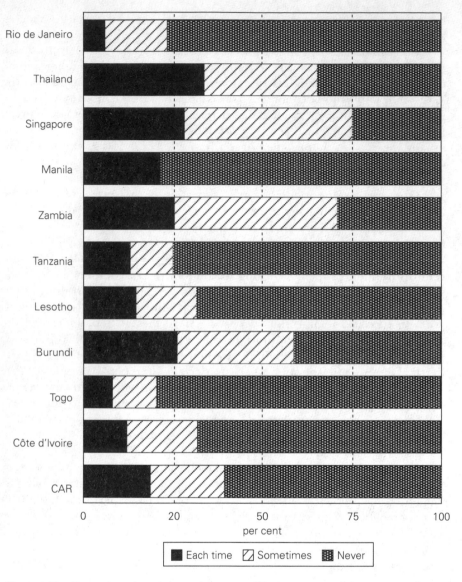

Figure 4.18: Frequency of condom use in commercial sex among men

levels of use were too low in most study sites. The denominator for the analyses was restricted to those who have heard of AIDS and who ever had sexual intercourse (virgins excluded). In Manila and Thailand, the levels of extra-marital sexual contact among women were less than two per cent and accordingly regressions were not conducted.

The results of the analyses are shown in Table 4.7 with the significant effects ($p < 0.05$) marked with one asterisk and interactive effects by an *x*.

Table 4.7: Summary of results of multiple regression analyses on reported risk behaviour

	Côte d'Ivoire	Burundi	Lusaka	Manila	Thailand	Rio de Janeiro
Among men						
Predictors						
Age	*	*	*	–	*	–
Education	*	*	–	–	*	–
Marital status	*	–	x	*	*	*
Residence	–	*	n	n	*	n
Personal vulnerability	*	–	x	–	*	*
Drinking habits	*	n	*	–	*	*
Among women						
Predictors						
Age	*	–	*	0	0	*
Education	*	–	–	0	0	*
Marital status	*	–	–	0	0	*
Residence	–	*	n	0	0	n
Personal vulnerability	*	*	–	0	0	*
Drinking habits	*	n	*	0	0	*

Notes: * Enters model as main effect (p < 0.05)
     x Enters model as interaction
     n Not included in country's data as predictor variable
     0 Not included as an outcome variable (number of cases too low)

Table 4.8: Net effects of age, education and marital status on proportion reporting risk behaviour in the last 12 months among sexually active men

	Adjusted proportions					
	Côte d'Ivoire	Burundi	Lusaka	Manila	Thailand	Rio de Janeiro
Age						
15–19	.57	.14	.41	NS	.62	NS
20–24	.60	.14	.59	NS	.40	NS
25–39	.55	.09	.38	NS	.31	NS
40–49	.42	.03	.21	NS	.28	NS
Education						
None	.41	.05	NS	NS	.28	NS
Primary	.47	.09	NS	NS	.28	NS
Secondary+	.61	.16	NS	NS	.41	NS
Marital status						
Currently	.47	NS	x	.07	.22	.31
Never	.73	NS	x	.50	.66	.77

Notes: x Interaction with personal vulnerability
     NS Variable not significant

Age is a predictor of risk behaviour in the three African sites, with the single exception of women in Burundi. In the non-African sites, age is not predictive of risk except in Thailand amongst men and in Rio de Janeiro amongst women.

The association between age and risk behaviour, after adjustment for other factors in the model, is shown for men in Table 4.8. In all four sites where age is a significant predictor, risk behaviour declines monotonically after age 25 years. Below this age, however, the pattern of association varies. In Côte d'Ivoire and Burundi, there is little or no difference between teenagers and young men aged 20 to 24. In Thailand the highest level of risk is found among those aged 15 to 19 years, while in Lusaka the 20 to 24 age group records the highest level of risk.

Significant associations between schooling and risk behaviour are less common than for age. Amongst men, significant net effects are found in only three out of six sites and amongst women, in only two out of four sites. In all cases, there is a positive association between risk behaviour and educational background. As shown in Table 4.8, there tends to be a large difference between those with secondary or higher schooling and the less educated.

Marital status enters the models as a main effect amongst men in five sites and in interaction with personal vulnerability in Lusaka. The magnitude of the association between marital status and non-regular sex can be seen in Table 4.8. In Manila, never-married men are seven times more likely to report such sexual contacts than those who are married; in Thailand, they are three times more likely and in Rio de Janeiro over twice as likely.

In Lusaka, an interaction effect indicates that for currently and formerly married men, higher personal vulnerability is associated with higher risk taking, but the opposite is found for never-married men. For women marital status emerges as a net predictor in only two of the six sites.

In the few surveys, where such a distinction is possible, there is no clear pattern regarding a link between urban/rural residence and risk behaviour. It is striking that the effect of urban/rural residence on risk behaviour, prominent in bivariate analysis, is so strongly attenuated or even disappears when other variables such as education and marital status are controlled. In Thailand and Côte d'Ivoire, unadjusted proportions of men reporting risk behaviour in urban versus rural settings were respectively .46 versus .28 and .56 versus .48. When adjusted, these proportions became .37 in urban Thailand versus .31 in rural, and .52 in both urban and rural Côte d'Ivoire. Amongst men in Burundi, the unadjusted proportions in urban and rural settings who reported risk behaviour were .12 and .07. After adjustment, the direction of the relationship changes, with values of .10 and .12, respectively; this difference is significant but clearly of little substantive importance.

In each of the four surveys where data on drinking habits were collected, men and women who reported regular drinking of alcohol had a greater probability of risk behaviour than those who did not take alcohol regularly. Both sexes in Manila and Thai women prove to be the exceptions here. Finally, perceived personal vulnerability to HIV/AIDS is associated with risk behaviour amongst men and women in Côte d'Ivoire, Lusaka and Rio de Janeiro and Thailand for men only. (The number of cases amongst women was too small for analysis.) Manila, again is the exception. Indeed Manila appears in many of the previous analyses as a rather atypical site, with only marital status amongst the six potential predictors entering the model. It suggests again that patterns of risk behaviour may be different in some Asian countries as compared to selected African sites.

Summary and Discussion

The findings presented here detail only a fraction of the vast amount of information on sexual behaviour that has been gathered in 15 populations through the WHO/GPA surveys. No doubt, there are limitations, some of which are imposed by the cross-national emphasis of the analysis. For instance, religious, ethnic, socio-economic and regional variations have been entirely omitted. Despite this, these survey findings are important for public health policy in many ways.

Levels of premarital sexual activity and rates of partner change among persons aged 15 to 19 years were shown to vary greatly between countries; clearly, sweeping generalizations about the high risk behaviour of young people are unwarranted. Differences between men and women in the proportions reporting sexual experience outside marriage in the last 12 months and in the number of non-marital partners were particularly marked in some populations. This polarization probably reflects the fact that young males have many of their sexual contacts with women involved in sex in exchange of money or gifts, a behaviour that, if unprotected, may carry enhanced risk of HIV infection.

Urban-rural disparities in proportions sexually active were less pronounced than expected and there was a strong correlation between behaviour in rural and urban areas. This result suggests that sexual behaviour among young people in cities and towns is still culturally linked to sexual behaviour in rural areas and that, with a few exceptions, risk behaviour is also present in rural areas. An additional independent predictor of sexual activity among youths was education: secondary schooling was associated with a substantial increase in risk behaviour among males, and primary schooling similarly associated amongst females. These results suggest that education can result in relaxation of social controls on behaviours in societies where such controls are still forceful. It reflects also a greater exposure to risk: the educated experience a longer span between puberty and first stable partnership.

A huge cross-cultural variability in the onset of sexual behaviour was demonstrated; in some societies over half of 15 year olds are already sexually experienced while, in others, nearly all are virgins at this age. There was no statistical association between female and male virginity at first marriage (or regular partnership), but a high level of virginity for women was found to be correlated with low levels of female extra-marital sex. This consistency may reflect a continuity of societal control on female sexuality.

The study populations also varied greatly in ages at which men and women first marry or enter a stable partnership. Contrary to the evidence of many demographic surveys, there was no clear evidence of increases in age at first stable partnership among the younger cohorts. Age differences between regular partners were between three and five years in most of the societies. Large age differences and early female age at marriage were associated with high levels of polygyny or of multiple partnerships. Levels of non-cohabitation among young married respondents were surprisingly high, especially in African surveys, where typically between one-fifth and one-third of men and women reported that they lived apart from their regular partner. As expected, there were significant associations between the level of non-cohabitation, the proportion of men reporting more than one regular female partner and the proportion reporting non-regular sex in the last year. This finding is important in demonstrating how the nature of the marital bond may influence sexual behaviour outside marriage.

The same comment applies to the low reported coital frequency among regular partners and to the unexpectedly large proportions of spouses who reported no sex during the last year or during the last month. Among the African surveys, between a quarter and a half reported no sex with a regular partner in the last month. Lactational taboos, polygyny, non-cohabitation and sex outside regular partnership may account for these low figures.

The prevalence of sex outside regular partnerships, if any, in the last year, ranges from less than 10 to nearly 50 per cent among males, but from 0 to less than 20 per cent among females. In all surveys, men were more likely to report non-marital sex and a higher number of sexual partners than women. There was a significant relationship between the level of premarital sex among adolescents and the level of non-regular sex among adults for both sexes, highlighting the existence of consistent cultural patterns of sexuality across the boundaries of age and marital status. The number of casual partners and the overall level of casual sex in a particular society were also correlated: there was a greater heterogeneity and larger numbers of people engaged in high risk behaviour when the proportion of people reporting non-regular sex was already high.

In some populations, sex in exchange of money and gifts represents an important part of sexual behaviour, while in others it plays only a marginal role. High levels of casual sex among men usually reduce the importance of commercial sex. Single or separated persons are more likely to engage in commercial sex than married ones. At the time of the surveys, condom use in such encounters was still uncommon for the great majority of men. Frequency of alcohol consumption was associated with the level of non-regular and commercial sex in most populations.

Logistic regressions to assess the simultaneous effects of age, education, marital status, residence and personal vulnerability on the likelihood of non-regular and commercial sex in the last 12 months showed that age and marital status were the most influential demographic predictors.

Although we must be cautious when interpreting self-reported data on sexual behaviour, the main descriptive results presented in this chapter show consistent patterns that should help to understand better levels of non-regular sex, the demographic correlates of sexual behaviour, and their relationships to the HIV pandemic. In this first cross-cultural attempt to examine aspects of sexual lifestyles, it has been consistently shown that broad generalizations about one particular population or region are misleading. No evidence was found of a universal trend towards earlier onset of sexual activity or towards later marriage or increased contact with sex workers. Gender, age and a few other demographic correlates were disclosed as powerful determinants of sexual behaviours in all populations though the strength of associations varied greatly between specific locations.

The analysis also emphasizes the need to relate specific components of behaviour to more general patterns of sexuality. Early age at sexual intercourse is not necessarily a risk factor if the first partner is or becomes a spouse. A low level of non-regular sex in a population may enhance HIV transmission if most sexual interactions are with sex workers and if condoms are not consistently used. Polygyny should not be regarded as conducive to HIV infection if polygyny is the rule and there are high levels of faithfulness within such unions. To be currently married or in a regular partnership is not necessarily linked to safe sex if cohabitation is not involved.

These necessary links argue for a broader definition of risk behaviours and to a greater sensitivity to gender considerations. Unless placed within their social and cultural context, isolated risk behaviours should not be considered as a sound basis for the extrapolation of the future course of the HIV pandemic. However, in populations where heterosexual intercourse is the main mode of HIV transmission, the monitoring of behavioural change through repeated surveys of the general population, should be an important part of the evaluation of AIDS control programmes (Johnson, *et al.*, 1992; ACSF, 1992; Mertens, *et al.*, 1994). At the same time, improvements in methods of data collection and the use of complementary methods involving qualitative studies are urgently needed.

Note

1   Translation: 'The exchange, a total phenomenon, is first a total exchange which includes food, manufacturing objects, and this most treasured category of goods, woman.'

Chapter 5

Condoms: Awareness, Attitudes and Use

Amir Mehryar

Introduction

Although primitive forms of the condom were employed as a means of pregnancy prevention over 3000 years ago (Finch and Green, 1963), its widespread use as an effective device for preventing sexually transmitted diseases
(STDs), particularly syphilis, during the past two centuries has made it highly
controversial (Tanquary and Witte, 1990). In many countries with the start
of the AIDS epidemic, the word *condom* has become a morally and emotion-
ally loaded term with connotations of illicit sex. As a result, and despite great
technological advances in the manufacture of inexpensive and reliable condoms during the second half of this century, their widespread use as a contraceptive has been hampered by their historical association with STD
prevention. Indeed, before the advent of AIDS, an avowed concern with
public morality and decency deterred some publicly funded family planning
organizations from openly promoting condoms, or making them available at
clinics. As a consequence, people seeking to use condoms had to overcome
physical constraints regarding availability and cost, as well as barriers of fear,
guilt and embarrassment associated with the taboo nature of the product.
Later developments of effective and convenient contraceptives for use by
women further undermined the need for the condom as a family planning
method.

Thus, when AIDS emerged as a global health problem in the mid-1980s
and the protective value of the condom against HIV was demonstrated, relatively small proportions of sexually active individuals in most countries were
using condoms as a contraceptive (Goldberg, *et al.*, 1989). In the late 1980s,
only about 45,000,000 married couples of reproductive age were using condoms as their main means of contraception. This figure accounts for about
5 per cent of couples in the reproductive age span and about 9 per cent of
all couples using some form of family planning (Liskin, *et al.*, 1990). Comparing these figures with the results of earlier surveys as documented in
Sherris, *et al.* (1982), the world-wide percentage of married couples using
condoms would seem to have changed little. At both times, the majority of
couples using condoms for family planning was living in developed countries.

Japan – where about 70 per cent of all family planning users and 45 per cent of all couples rely on condoms – accounts for almost 20 per cent of all married couples using condoms as a contraceptive. In Scandinavian countries, over 20 per cent of married women of reproductive age rely on condom use by their partners for family planning. In most other developed countries with the necessary data, 5 to 15 per cent of women of reproductive age use condoms for pregnancy prevention. Somewhat higher proportions of couples practising family planning are known to be using the condom as their main means of protection in such rapidly developing Asian, Latin American, and Caribbean countries as Hong Kong (32 per cent), Grenada (26 per cent), Trinidad and Tobago (22 per cent), Costa Rica (19 per cent), Taiwan (18 per cent), and Jamaica (16 per cent). Even in Pakistan, where only 8 per cent of married couples were using any method of contraception, condom users accounted for 22 per cent of all contraceptors in 1984–5. By contrast, in some of the largest developing countries with contraceptive prevalence rates of 66 per cent or more (e.g. China, Thailand, and Brazil) only 3 per cent or less of all contraceptors were known to be using condoms as their main means of pregnancy prevention. In sub-Saharan Africa, where contraceptive prevalence rates are generally lower than in most developing countries, very small proportions of modern contraceptive users are known to rely on condoms as their main means of family planning. Even in Botswana, Kenya and Zimbabwe where relatively large proportions (30–45 per cent) of eligible couples surveyed report contraceptive practice, only about 1 per cent were condom users in the late 1980s.

With the recognition of AIDS as a global public health problem, the need to promote condoms as a means of protection against HIV and other STDs became an urgent priority. As mentioned earlier, condoms have a long history as an effective means of STD and pregnancy prevention. Their effectiveness against HIV has also been demonstrated (Conant, *et al.*, 1986; Van de Perre and Sprecher-Golderberger, 1987; Feldbum and Fortney, 1988; Rietmeijer, *et al.*, 1988; Fathallah, 1990; Liskin, *et al.*, 1990). Field studies have confirmed the effectiveness of condoms in reducing the chances of HIV infection in such groups as sex workers and their clients, homosexual and bisexual men, male and female drug injectors, and sexually active couples one of whom is known to be HIV infected (Mann, *et al.*, 1986; American Public Health Association, 1988; Ngugi, *et al.*, 1988; Wilkins, *et al.*, 1989; Kamenga, *et al.*, 1989). Consequently, the promotion of condom use has been adopted as a general policy by all international health organizations and by most National AIDS Control Programmes.

Open and vigorous promotion of condoms as the most practical means of prevention of HIV and other STDs, however, has faced covert resistance by many policymakers and has been overtly opposed by certain influential religious groups in many countries. These objections are usually rooted in the historical association of the condom with illicit sex and STDs. But in view of the fatal nature of AIDS and the global support for its prevention, opponents of the condom usually find it necessary to express their objections in more socially acceptable and defensible terms. Thus, in several developing countries seriously threatened by the AIDS pandemic, political authorities have been reluctant to support wide-scale condom promotion campaigns by claiming that condoms are not sufficiently effective at preventing HIV infection and may prove too expensive in the long run. In other countries, the open promotion of condoms by the mass media and their inclusion in educational programmes have been discouraged on the grounds that public discussion of condoms may encourage sexual promiscuity, especially among young people. In still other countries, particularly in Africa, condom promotion campaigns have not received adequate support either from politicians or public opinion leaders because of an untested belief that condoms, being foreign to the local culture, have little chance of being accepted or used by African men.

Measurement of Variables

In view of the controversies surrounding the condom and its potential importance for AIDS prevention and the dearth of scientific data regarding its acceptability and use in most developing countries, social and behavioural scientists working with WHO/GPA and National AIDS Control Programmes were urged to consider condoms as a priority research topic. To assist such research and facilitate the collection of cross-nationally comparable data on condoms, it was decided to include a section on condom awareness and use in the standard KABP and PR questionnaires developed by WHO/GPA.

In the KABP questionnaire, the section on condoms starts with a general question asking respondents to name all contraceptive methods that they have heard of. If the condom is not mentioned in response to this general question, the following brief description is offered: *Men can wear a rubber or condom during sex to prevent pregnancy* and the respondent is then asked *Have you heard of this method?* Those who indicate an awareness of the condom are asked, *Have you ever used a condom?* Respondents who have indicated an awareness of AIDS in answer to earlier questions are also asked whether, and which, of the contraceptives they had mentioned can be used to avoid getting AIDS. This question is followed by two specific questions on sources of condom supply in their community, and the latter's approximate distance (in travel time) from their place of residence or work. *Do you know of any place or person where you could get condoms? IF YES, Where would you go if you wanted to get some?* and *How long would it take you to go to this place or person to get condoms?*

In the PR questionnaire, the section on condoms starts with a general question on knowledge of methods of contraception. After recording respondents' spontaneous answers to this question, the interviewer reads out the names of all contraceptives not mentioned by the respondent, describes them briefly and asks if the respondent knows that method. For each method known, the respondent is asked: *Have you or your spouse or regular partner ever used this method?* And for each method ever used, they are asked, *Are you or your partner currently using this method?* These questions are followed by the two questions on sources of condom supply and their perceived distance.

In both KABP and PR surveys, respondents were further asked to reveal their perceptions of, and attitudes towards, the condom by expressing their agreement or disagreement with ten statements about condoms. This topic was introduced in the following manner: *People say many things about condoms. I am going to read some of the things they say. Listen carefully and tell me whether you agree or disagree with each of the statements I read out.* To avoid forcing respondents to make *agree* or *disagree* response, they were provided with a third response alternative of *Uncertain, Do not know.* The ten statements are as follows:

- Condoms are good at preventing pregnancy if used properly.
- Condoms make sex less enjoyable.
- Condoms are most appropriate for use with casual sex partners.
- Condoms are easy to use.
- Condom use is against my religion.
- Condoms are offensive to husbands/wives/regular sexual partners.
- Condoms can climb up into the womb or stomach.
- The price of condoms is too high to use regularly.
- Condoms can prevent venereal diseases if used properly.
- Condoms are most appropriate for use with spouse or a regular partner.

The same ten statements were included in both types of model questionnaire although the order of questions was not constant. It may also be worth noting that, in the KABP instrument, questions concerning the condom were asked after two long sections on AIDS knowledge, whereas in PR surveys, questions on AIDS came after the condom section.

This chapter summarizes findings on awareness, use and attitudes to the condom collected through the questions described above. There are several additional questions on condoms in other sections of the KABP and PR questionnaires. For example, in the section on the relationship between behaviour and AIDS of the KABP questionnaire, respondents who indicate a belief that AIDS could be prevented by behaviour change are asked to specify the kinds of behaviour change that could protect them against AIDS. *Condom use* is one of the coded alternatives. Respondents who fail to mention condoms in response to this question are asked if they believe that the condom can protect them against AIDS. In the PR questionnaire, too, respondents are asked if they used a condom during any commercial sex encounters over the previous 12 months. These results are merely summarized in this chapter because they have been discussed in Chapter 4.

Awareness of Condoms and Access to Supplies

As mentioned above, condom awareness was measured in two ways. First, through a general, open-ended question, on methods that men use to avoid making their spouse/partner pregnant. Second, if the above question did not elicit the term *condom* (or any of its local variants) as one of the response alternatives, a simple definition of the condom was read out followed by the direct probe: *Have you heard of a condom?* Obviously, the two approaches rely on rather different cognitive processes (i.e., recall versus recognition) and may reflect quite different levels of awareness or knowledge. In this part of the analysis, however, all respondents who mentioned condom spontaneously or claimed familiarity with it in answer to further probing will be considered as having some knowledge of condoms and their potential uses.

Figure 5.1 summarizes the level of condom awareness or knowledge as defined above separately for men and women in the 14 research sites with the necessary data. (Condom awareness questions were omitted from the schedule used in Sri Lanka.) It is immediately apparent that the proportion of respondents who knew of condoms varied considerably from one research site to another. Thus, in some sites almost everyone knew about condoms, while in other sites over 50 per cent of respondents had not yet heard of them. The lowest levels of condom awareness were found in the four African countries (Côte d'Ivoire, Central African Republic, Togo, and Burundi) and the highest levels in South East Asia (Thailand and Singapore) and in Rio de Janeiro. The remarkably low level of condom awareness (62 per cent) reported by the Manila sample as well as the relatively high awareness revealed by respondents in such African sites as Lusaka (77 per cent), and Tanzania (72 per cent), however, indicate that non-awareness of condoms is by no means confined to Africa. The apparent unfamiliarity shown by Manila respondents is surprising both in comparison with other Asian samples and with regard to the high level of education of the Manila sample. This is also true of the relatively low level of condom awareness displayed by women in Rio de Janeiro, where 45 per cent of the total sample have secondary education or higher. More men than women have heard of the condom in all 14 research sites but the differences are not very large in most instances. In only seven of the 14 research sites did the male/female difference in condom awareness exceed 10 per cent. The largest such differences occurred in Côte d'Ivoire (25 per cent), Central African Republic (16 per cent), Burundi (15 per cent), Manila (16 per cent), Mauritius (16 per cent) and Guinea Bissau (10 per cent).

Although women in general tend to be in a disadvantaged position with regard to such important indicators of modernization as level of education and exposure to mass media, their lower awareness of condoms does not seem to be entirely due to such factors. In the overwhelming majority of cases, women and men of the same educational level, the same degree of media exposure, and the same residential status (urban vs rural) show the

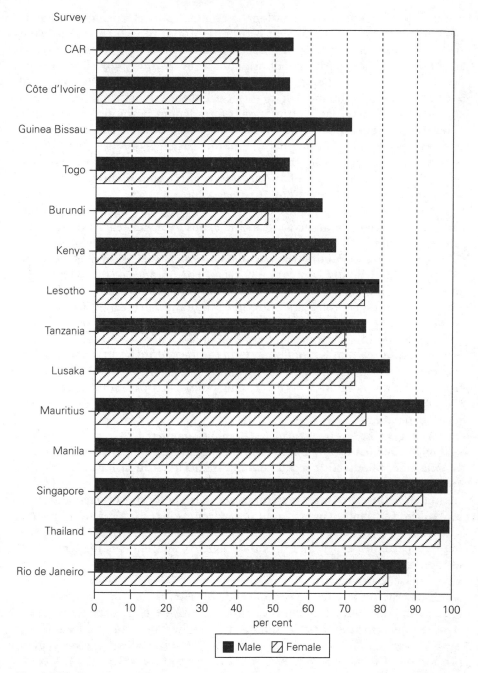

Figure 5.1: Percentage of all males and females who were aware of condoms

same disparity in terms of condom awareness. This is not entirely unexpected, but the fact remains that large proportions of women (27 per cent to 71 per cent) in sub-Saharan African countries included in these surveys had not yet heard of the condom at the time of the study. Even in the cosmopolitan city of Manila, 45 per cent of women sampled (as compared with 29 per cent of the men) had not heard of the condom. Clearly, women should be considered as a prime target for condom promotion campaigns. Their relative ignorance of the condom might not be a serious disadvantage in the case of family planning because of the existence of more effective and convenient alternatives. But the situation is quite different in the case of HIV and STDs, and women can ill afford to leave the responsibility for knowing, obtaining and using the condom to their male partners.

Awareness of condoms was analyzed by respondents' age, marital status, education, place of residence and media exposure. With regard to age, one would hope for high levels of condom awareness among people aged 15 to 19 years who are beginning their sexual careers, as well as among the sexually active young adults aged 20 to 39 years. The findings of the WHO/GPA surveys are rather disappointing with regard to the youngest age group who display the lowest condom awareness in eight of the 14 research sites and the second lowest condom awareness rates in four others. In only one country (Thailand), do they have the highest level of awareness. Interestingly, young women would seem to be somewhat better informed than older women, but the same is not true for men. Thus, while male teenagers have the second highest condom awareness levels in only one country (Central African Republic), their female counterparts occupy the first or second position in four study populations.

As expected, levels of formal schooling completed by respondents are strongly associated with condom awareness in all research sites. In 11 of the 14 sites respondents with secondary and higher education have the highest condom awareness, and those with no schooling the lowest. The only substantial deviations from this general pattern are rather unexpected and hard to explain. In Manila, higher condom awareness is recorded among people with primary education (72 per cent) than those with secondary and higher schooling (61 per cent); and in Rio de Janeiro, awareness is higher among women with no schooling (88 per cent) than among those with primary education (72 per cent).

Similarly, the urban–rural differential in awareness conforms to expectations. In nine out of the ten research sites with both urban and rural samples, the urban group has substantially higher levels of condom awareness than the rural. The only exception is Lesotho where a slightly higher proportion of rural respondents (78 per cent) than the urban (74 per cent) had heard of condoms.

While awareness of condoms is a logical precondition for their use, knowledge of a source of supply within reasonable travelling time is a prerequisite, in normal circumstances, for the purchase of condoms. Accordingly,

Table 5.1: Main source of condom supply mentioned by respondents who have heard of condoms

Survey	Shop	Chemist Pharmacy	Health Centre	F.P. Office	Other	None Known	Total	N
		Main Source of Condom Supply (per cent)						
CAR	2	31	38	3	2	24	100	1145
Côte d'Ivoire	–	62	9	2	4	22	100	1240
Guinea Bissau	–	26	15	40	17	1	100	874
Togo	1	34	37	17	5	4	100	1175
Burundi	1	27	28	–	3	41	100	1299
Kenya	–	12	3	63	4	18	100	1866
Lesotho	1	12	44	24	2	17	100	1213
Lusaka	11	41	16	1	1	30	100	1536
Mauritius	4	55	10	19	10	–	100	2069
Manila	2	49	30	4	4	11	100	1000
Singapore	55	11	23	–	1	9	100	2011
Thailand	–	16	22	23	–	39	100	2733
Rio de Janeiro	4	86	1	1	1	7	100	1130

respondents who reported knowledge of condoms were asked whether they knew of a source where they could be obtained and, if so, what type of place they would visit to obtain supplies. In a sub-set of surveys, they were further asked about the distance to this source.

Table 5.1 shows the main, or preferred, source of condoms mentioned by respondents. The first point to note is that appreciable minorities of those aware of condoms were unable to mention any place where supplies could be obtained. In five of the 13 surveys available for analysis, about one in five respondents were ignorant of any source. This proportion rises to 30 per cent in Lusaka, a surprising result in view of the fact that Lusaka is a capital city. The lowest level of knowledge is found in Burundi where 41 per cent were unaware of a source. At the other extreme, 90 per cent, or thereabouts, of men and women aware of condoms were also aware of a supply source in Guinea Bissau, Togo, Manila and Singapore. The results for Guinea Bissau and Togo should be interpreted cautiously though, because large proportions of those claiming to know a source of supply were unable to estimate the travelling time (Table 5.2). This discrepancy suggests that the question on knowledge of source may have been misunderstood or that such knowledge is very superficial.

In terms of the types of sources mentioned by respondents, the main interest lies in the huge variations in the relative importance of private commercial outlets (shops, pharmacies) and public sector health and family planning centres. In the metropolitan surveys, commercial outlets, not surprisingly, are dominant. In Côte d'Ivoire and Mauritius, this is also true. In Kenya, Guinea Bissau, Lesotho and Thailand, on the other hand, respondents were much more likely to mention a health or family planning centre than a shop or pharmacy. In the case of Kenya and Thailand, well developed family planning services help to account for this pattern. In Guinea Bissau

Table 5.2: Among respondents who know a source of condoms, per cent distribution according to travelling time to that source

Survey	<15	15–29	30–59	60+	DK	Total	N
			Minutes				
CAR	17	27	21	34	2	100	866
Côte d'Ivoire	49	20	14	5	12	100	963
Guinea Bissau	13	7	10	11	60	100	869
Togo		–35–		15	50	100	1122
Lusaka	32	1	1	61	7	100	1080
Mauritius	23	29	26	3	19	100	2069
Thailand	44	12	11	4	30	100	2250
Rio de Janeiro	81	17	2	0	1	100	1052

and Lesotho, the salience of public sector sources of supply may reflect a poorly developed commercial market.

Table 5.2 shows the reported travelling time to the preferred condom source, among those aware of any source. As already mentioned, large proportions of respondents in Guinea Bissau and Togo (60 and 50 per cent respectively) were unable to give the travelling time. In Thailand and Mauritius also, appreciable minorities could not answer this question.

With regard to proximity to a source, Rio de Janeiro is easily the most advantaged site; four out of five respondents were within 15 minutes of the condom outlet. The situation appears to be very different in the other metropolitan site, Lusaka, where a suspiciously high proportion (61 per cent) reported that the nearest condom source was one hour or more away from their home or place of work.

An attempt to summarize the components of condom knowledge and access is made in Figure 5.2. The left-hand segment of each bar represents the percentage of all respondents who are unaware of condoms and the next segment those who have heard of condoms but know no source. In five of the African sites, the sum of these two proportions accounts for over half of the entire sample. Thus in the Central African Republic, Côte d'Ivoire, Guinea Bissau, Togo and Burundi, over half of all men and women were faced in the late 1980s with insufficient knowledge to be able to use condoms. In Kenya, Lesotho and Lusaka, this knowledge is somewhat higher. Between 43 per cent (Lusaka females) and 68 per cent (Lesotho males) were aware of condoms and a source. In the non-African populations, knowledge of condoms and sources tends to be higher still. Large majorities of men and women in Rio de Janeiro, Singapore and Thailand knew where to obtain condoms, with somewhat lower levels in Mauritius and Manila. Claimed knowledge of a source may be insufficient for positive motives to be translated into appropriate behaviour if sources are so unfamiliar that respondents are unable to estimate how long it would take to reach them, or if the travelling time is long. Accordingly, the right-hand two segments of the bars in Figure 5.2 represent the percentages of all respondents who live (or work) within 30

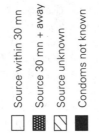

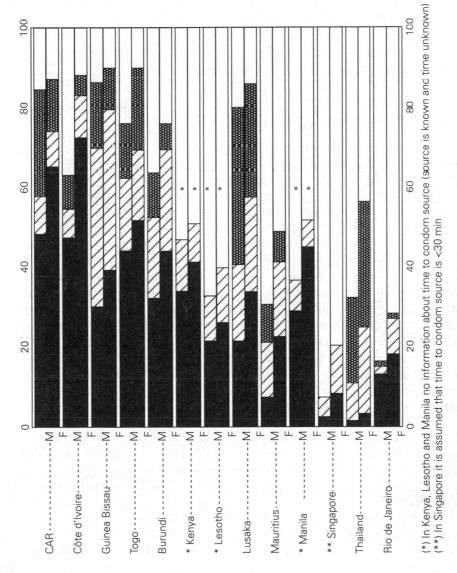

(*) In Kenya, Lesotho and Manila no information about time to condom source (source is known and time unknown)
(**) In Singapore it is assumed that time to condom source is <30 min

Figure 5.2: A summary of condom access among men and women

minutes of the nearest source and those who do not. As noted earlier, the relevant information to make this distinction was collected in only nine of the 13 surveys. In two cases, the absence of data does not represent a serious omission. In Manila and Singapore, it can be assumed that the majority of those aware of a source live or work within a short distance of it. In Kenya and Lesotho, however, this assumption is clearly invalid.

A clear-cut African, non-African divide is apparent in terms of access to condoms. In most of the African surveys, only small minorities of all respondents are classified as having good access to condoms (i.e. aware of a source within 30 minutes travelling time). For men, the relevant percentages are 15, 17, 21, 25, 37 and 38 for the Central African Republic, Guinea Bissau, Togo (where the distinction is 60 rather than 30 minutes), Lusaka, Burundi and Côte d'Ivoire, respectively. The corresponding figures for women are even lower. There clearly remains a major task of promoting condom knowledge and increasing access in many African countries.

Condom Use

Although awareness of condoms is essential for their initial trial, many factors determine the ultimate adoption and consistent use of the condom by those who already know of them. Among these, sexual activity is the logically most relevant factor. Another important determinant of condom use, a felt need for protection against unwanted pregnancy or STDs, also depends on being sexually active.

Two major forms of condom use are usually distinguished: ever-used and current use. While the PR instrument measures current use, both types of questionnaires were designed to measure whether or not condoms had ever been used. The prevalence of ever-use may be based on several different denominators: all respondents; all respondents aware of condoms; all sexually active respondents; and all respondents who are defined by some criterion to be in need of condom use.

Each of these ratios has its own particular use and meaning. The proportion of condom users in the whole adult sample provides a broad summary measure of the life time prevalence of condom use. As not all adults are sexually active or in need of protection, this ratio should be interpreted as an underestimate of the population that may in fact be protected against either unwanted pregnancy or sexually transmitted diseases. The second measure of condom use, that is the ratio of condom users to those who have heard of condoms, gives a more realistic picture of the prevalence of condom use in that it takes into account only that section of the population who has already heard of the condom and presumably has some idea of its characteristics and potential costs and benefits. The third measure of condom ever-use, based on sexually active persons, provides a more valid estimate of the likelihood of protection against unwanted pregnancy, HIV/AIDS and

Table 5.3: *Percentage who have ever used condoms: summary statistics based on different denominators*

| | Denominators | | |
	Total Sample	Those aware of condoms	Sexually active respondents
Males			
Median	20.0	38.0	24.3
Range	7.6–39.6	17.9–51.8	12.2–65.8
Females			
Median	8.4	16.0	9.3
Range	5.4–29.6	7.3–34.2	5.9–50.7
All			
Median	13.6	26.4	19.8
Range	8.9–34.3	14.1–45.0	10.2–58.0

other STDs. Because of their common numerator, the three indices of condom use are closely correlated, the size of the correlation varying according to the levels of condom awareness and sexual activity in the sample. Similarly the relative standing of different research sites with regard to condom ever-use remains more or less the same regardless of which rate is used.

The proportions of all men and women who have ever used condoms are shown in Figure 5.3. For men, this proportion ranges from 8 to 40 per cent, with a median value of 20 per cent. For women, the corresponding median is only 8 per cent with a range of 5 to 30 per cent. As seen in Table 5.3, the median proportions who have ever used condoms doubles for both males and females when persons unaware of condoms are removed from the denominator; however the range of values among the study populations does not narrow, indicating that knowledge itself cannot account for the variability of condom use across these societies. For instance, in Côte d'Ivoire, 45 per cent of all those aware of condoms have tried them, whereas in Burundi, Kenya, Lesotho and Tanzania less than 18 per cent have done so. When condom users are calculated as a percentage of all sexually active persons, the medians revert to values close to those based on entire samples, but the upper end of the range rises dramatically. In Mauritius, Singapore and Thailand over half of all sexually active men have used condoms. The corresponding figures for women are 36, 51 and 22 per cent, respectively. Figure 5.3 (based on entire samples) indicates that ever-use of condoms is particularly low in Africa where, in five study populations (Togo, Burundi, Kenya, Lesotho and Tanzania), 10 per cent or less of all respondents report ever having used a condom; the levels fall short of 20 per cent in another two countries (Central African Republic and Côte d'Ivoire). Only in Guinea Bissau (24 per cent) and Lusaka (27 per cent) do one quarter to one third of all respondents report ever using a condom. Of the six research sites outside continental Africa, four (Mauritius, Singapore, Thailand and Rio de Janeiro)

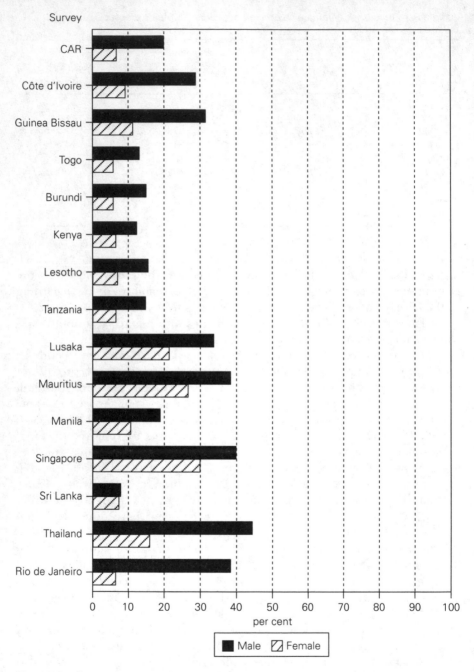

Figure 5.3:   Percentage of all males and females who have ever used condoms

have relatively high condom ever-use rates, whereas two others (Manila and Sri Lanka) fall just above the median (13.6 per cent) level for all 15 sites.

The overall low levels of condom use in the majority of African sites are in line with results of family planning surveys conducted in sub-Saharan Africa (Sherris, *et al.*, 1982; London, *et al.*, 1985; Ross, *et al.*, 1988; Goldberg, *et al.*, 1989; Liskin, *et al.*, 1990). The higher levels of condom use reported in Lusaka may reflect the fact that the Lusaka sample includes an over-representation of the highly educated (58 per cent with secondary or higher schooling). The high condom use reported in Guinea Bissau is more difficult to explain particularly because of the relatively low levels of urbanization (37 per cent), education (46 per cent with no schooling), and media exposure (only 10 per cent with high media exposure rating) that characterize this sample. On the other hand, the low condom use rates reported in Sri Lanka and Manila are surprising in view of the advanced level of modernization of these two south-east Asian societies and their long history of family planning. The findings, however, are consistent with results of other surveys conducted in the Philippines and Sri Lanka. According to data summarized by Liskin, *et al.* (1990), only 1 per cent and 2 per cent of married women of reproductive age were using condoms in the mid-1980s as their main method of contraception in Philippines and Sri Lanka. This was despite the fact that 45 per cent and 62 per cent of married women of reproductive age of these two countries were using a method, and over one-fifth of them a male method of contraception. Moreover, contraceptive prevalence surveys carried out in the Philippines in 1978 and 1986 indicate that the proportion of couples using the condom had decreased by more than two-thirds during this period (Liskin, *et al.*, 1990).

In all research sites, men are more likely to have tried a condom than women, a not unexpected result in view of the fact that condoms may be widely used as a means of protection against STDs. The largest male–female difference in condom use is found in Rio de Janeiro where only 9 per cent of sexually experienced women compared with 46 per cent of men report use of a condom. The differences between men and women are also striking in the Central African Republic, Côte d'Ivoire, Guinea Bissau, Togo, Burundi, Lesotho and Thailand where men reporting condom use outnumber women by a factor of two or more to one. In Kenya too, the ratio of male to female condom use is just under 2. At the other extreme, the smallest male–female differences in condom use among the sexually experienced belong to Sri Lanka (1.1 per cent) and Singapore (1.3 per cent). It may be of some interest to note that these two research sites occupy the two extremes of the condom use rates revealed by the present surveys. Despite these differences, there is a moderately high degree of positive association between the relative positions of different research sites with regard to condom use rates of men and women. This is indicated by a Spearman rank correlation coefficient of .63.

The gender differentials, favouring men, in reported condom use hold across all age groups, all three marital statuses, and high risk behaviours.

They also persist across different levels of media exposure, education, and urban/rural residence. The few exceptions to these generalizations are small in size and are not statistically significant.

These and other differentials in ever-use of condoms are shown in Table 5.4. Because of large differences in sexual experience by age, marital status and education, the denominator in this table excludes persons who have never had sexual intercourse. It might be expected that experience of condoms would rise with age, simply because of cumulative lifetime exposure to opportunity and need. In fact, the opposite pattern emerges. The oldest age group has the lowest condom use in all but four sites. This pattern indicates that, in most research sites, condom use, as with other methods of contraception, is a relatively recent innovation. The strikingly high condom use reported by young men aged 15 to 24 years in comparison with the very low use among the oldest age groups in such African sites as the Central African Republic, Côte d'Ivoire, Burundi, and Lusaka may be a reflection of the success of anti-AIDS campaigns undertaken recently in persuading sexually active young people to try condoms. The lack of difference between older and younger age groups in countries with a longer history of family planning and/or a higher prevalence of contraception (e.g. Guinea-Bissau, Kenya, Mauritius, Singapore, Thailand and Rio de Janeiro), lends partial support to this interpretation.

It is encouraging to observe that the youngest age groups (15–19 and 20–24 years) compare favourably with other age cohorts in most research sites in terms of condom ever-use. Nevertheless, the absolute number of sexually experienced young men and women who report having ever used a condom in the majority of research sites – particularly in sub-Saharan Africa – are too small to be adequate for the challenge posed by the AIDS pandemic. The problem is particularly serious in the case of sexually active young women of whom less than 16 per cent have ever tried a condom in 11 of the 15 research sites.

If condoms were used mainly for family planning purposes, one would expect the currently married and formerly married segments of the population to report higher condom use. This is the case in only Mauritius and Sri Lanka. In the ten other study populations, the never-married have the highest level of reported condom use. The relatively high reported rates of condom use among the never-married sexually active respondents supports the conclusion reached above regarding the recent origin of condom use in most research sites, particularly in Africa.

As expected, there is a close association between reported condom use and level of schooling. People with secondary and higher education were more likely to report condom use than the less educated in all 14 research sites. The same general pattern is observed for both men and women, except in Manila where women with no education have the highest condom use. Similarly, larger proportions of urban respondents than those from rural areas report ever having used a condom.

Condoms: Awareness, Attitudes and Use

Table 5.4(a): Percentage of sexually experienced men who have ever used condoms, by background characteristics

Characteristics	CAR	Côte d'Ivoire	Guinea Bissau	Togo	Burundi	Kenya	Lesotho	Tanzania	Lusaka	Mauritius	Manila	Singapore	Sri Lanka	Thailand	Rio de Janeiro
Age:															
15–19	34	42	46	9	18	10	23	14	55	30	37	62	19	56	37
20–24	34	45	50	18	29	28	17	11	59	34	29	59	16	55	47
25–39	16	33	47	17	21	18	19	17	38	50	24	69	12	55	41
40–49	11	13	20	12	9	17	10	12	15	64	21	63	11	42	32
50+	12	3	7	12	–	2	9	10	3	48	19	–	–	–	–
Marital Status:															
Currently	18	30	30	15	17	16	13	14	33	53	19	64	12	48	37
Formerly	16	29	38	17	50	3	62	9	35	55	44	20	–	46	71
Never	37	34	50	11	21	20	26	20	52	39	37	77	11	68	43
Residence:															
Urban	35	40	47	26	26	27	19	21	–	51	–	–	16	71	–
Rural	15	19	26	10	8	13	14	6	–	51	–	–	10	44	–
Education:															
None	6	6	10	4	8	2	15	6	8	32	–	50	–	21	30
Primary	15	22	29	15	13	13	15	13	27	51	17	54	–	41	29
Secondary+	42	51	64	26	46	23	18	28	43	53	25	71	–	73	50
Media Exposure:															
Low	11	6	14	7	6	–	11	7	26	37	18	64	4	33	38
Medium	31	26	49	21	24	–	20	21	40	44	20	59	10	50	30
High	51	50	78	40	44	–	23	46	49	56	26	68	14	69	44
Risk Behaviour:															
Yes	40	47	46	25	52	25	18	–	67	50	49	94	43	74	51
No	18	20	23	12	15	12	13	–	28	50	19	62	11	42	36
Total	21.0	30.3	33.0	14.8	18.5	16.4	16.1	14.0	36.3	50.8	24.3	65.8	12.2	52.3	39.8

Table 5.4(b): Percentage of sexually experienced women who have used condoms, by background characteristics

Characteristics	CAR	Côte d'Ivoire	Guinea Bissau	Togo	Burundi	Kenya	Lesotho	Tanzania	Lusaka	Mauritius	Manila	Singapore	Sri Lanka	Thailand	Rio de Janeiro
Age:															
15–19	10	16	21	8	11	11	9	5	31	25	12	33	9	13	15
20–24	8	15	11	9	10	12	7	10	29	31	12	43	14	20	12
25–39	5	7	14	6	8	9	10	10	20	44	18	54	13	26	7
40–49	3	1	4	2	4	6	5	8	14	44	19	47	7	13	5
50+	–	–	–	3	–	3	5	2	–	11	15	–	–	–	–
Marital Status:															
Currently	6	9	9	6	7	8	7	8	23	39	18	51	11	22	6
Formerly	5	5	30	3	19	4	–	13	21	15	12	39	5	15	9
Never	13	15	27	3	9	12	12	21	35	–	23	33	4	9	16
Residence:															
Urban	12	13	20	8	12	21	10	12	–	37	–	–	14	34	–
Rural	3	5	7	5	3	6	7	2	–	34	–	–	9	16	–
Education:															
None	2	2	5	3	5	4	7	3	10	24	33	35	–	7	5
Primary	9	11	12	9	8	8	4	10	13	35	17	48	–	18	4
Secondary+	20	26	29	17	16	15	14	21	36	46	17	55	–	41	11
Media Exposure:															
Low	3	4	7	5	6	–	5	6	16	26	10	37	6	15	12
Medium	15	14	25	11	10	–	8	13	31	29	18	51	10	22	4
High	35	24	23	11	23	–	34	30	38	44	18	52	13	34	8
Risk Behaviour:															
Yes	18	27	21	12	39	17	8	–	64	–	36	–	–	37	17
No	6	7	10	6	6	7	8	–	22	36	17	51	11	21	7
Total	6.8	9.3	12.3	5.9	7.3	8.7	8.0	8.5	24.2	35.8	17.4	50.7	10.8	21.5	7.5

In all 14 research sites with the necessary data, individuals that have reported engagement in sexual intercourse outside of regular partnerships in the last 12 months are more likely to have used condoms than other individuals. With only two exceptions, this difference applies to both male and female respondents.

Thus far, we have established that ever-use of condoms varies substantially according to the demographic and social circumstances and the sexual behaviour of individuals. For instance, experience of condoms appears to be more common among the young, the sexually active unmarried, the urban and more educated than among other subgroups. In order to explore these relationships further, logistic regression analysis was carried out on a sub-set of six surveys. A total of nine regressor variables was chosen. These include the four socio-demographic factors (age, education, marital status and residence), a behavioural variable, a variable that summarizes exposure to information about AIDS and three cognitive or attitudinal variables. The latter include perceived personal risk of HIV infection, belief in sexual transmission and perceived severity of AIDS. The precise definitions of these and other variables may be found in Chapter 2. This analysis was performed for sexually experienced respondents who had heard of AIDS and was done separately for men and women.

The results of the logistic regression are summarized in Table 5.5 which identifies predictor variables that have a significant (p < 0.05) net effect on reported condom use. As part of the analysis, all first-order interactions were systematically assessed. Table 5.5 also shows those predictors that have a significant interactive effect on condom use. Perhaps the single most important result is the strong net association between reported risk behaviour in the last 12 months and ever-use of condoms. Table 5.6 show the difference in ever-use of condoms between respondents who reported sex outside regular partnerships and those who did not, after adjustment for the other regressor variables. Not only is the relationship statistically significant for all groups except Thai women, but it is very strong. Typically, male respondents who reported risk behaviour are nearly twice as likely to have tried condoms as those reporting no risk. Among Rio de Janeiro males, risk behaviour interacts with education. Unexpectedly, the association between sexual behaviour and condom use is very strong among the uneducated, but not significant for those with primary or secondary schooling.

For females, the link between risk behaviour and condom use is even more pronounced than for males, though the number of women reporting any sexual intercourse outside the marriage or regular partnerships is very small in some surveys. In Burundi, for instance, women who report non-regular sex are over four times as likely to have tried condoms as others, and in Rio de Janeiro they are over three times as likely.

With regard to age, the logistic regression confirms the results of the bivariate analysis. Current age has a significant main effect among all study groups except for Manila and Rio de Janeiro, and among Burundi males. For

Table 5.5: *Summary of results of logistic regression analyses on ever-use of condoms*

Predictors	Males					
	Côte d'Ivoire	Burundi	Lusaka	Manila	Thailand	Rio de Janeiro
Age	*	*	*	–	*	–
Education	*	*	*	–	x	x
Marital status	x	x	–	*	–	*
Residence	x	*	na	na	x	na
Belief in sexual transmission	na	–	–	–	–	–
Reported risk behaviour	*	*	*	*	*	x
Information exposure	na	*	*	–	na	na
Perceived severity	na	–	–	–	na	na
Personal vulnerability	*	–	–	–	–	*
Interaction: age by marital status	–	*	–	–	–	–
Interaction: residence by marital status	*	–	na	na	–	na
Interaction: education by residence	–	–	na	na	*	na

Predictors	Females					
	Côte d'Ivoire	Burundi	Lusaka	Manila	Thailand	Rio de Janeiro
Age	*	*	*	–	*	–
Education	*	–	x	–	x	*
Marital status	*	–	*	–	–	–
Residence	–	*	na	na	*	na
Belief in sexual transmission	na	–	*	–	–	–
Reported risk behaviour	*	*	*	*	–	*
Information exposure	na	*	–	–	na	na
Perceived severity	na	–	–	–	na	na
Personal vulnerability	–	–	x	–	–	–
Interaction: Education by personal vulnerability	–	–	*	–	–	–

Notes: * Enters model as main variable (p < 0.05)
  x Enters model as an interaction
  na Data not available

the latter group, there is an age–marital status interaction; generally, condom use is higher among young people, except for men aged 15 to 19 years who have never been married or had a regular partner. The effects of age are particularly pronounced in Côte d'Ivoire and Lusaka as shown in terms of adjusted percentages who have ever tried condoms (Table 5.4). The common pattern is one of a little difference between the two youngest age groups. Thereafter, there is a steep downwards gradient. In Thailand, however, the relationship between age and condom use is quite different. For both men and women, highest use is found at intermediate ages.

The earlier bivariate analysis suggested that ever-use of condoms was

Table 5.6: Net effects of reported sexual behaviour on use of condom

| | Adjusted percentage who have ever used | | | |
| | Males | | Females | |
Survey	Risk Behaviour	No Risk Behaviour	Risk Behaviour	No Risk Behaviour
Côte d'Ivoire	38	23	21	8
Burundi	39	16	37	8
Lusaka	51	36	39	27
Manila	41	20	42	16
Thailand	71	44	22	22
Rio de Janeiro	x	x	21	6

x   Interactive effect

Table 5.7: Net effects of respondents' age on use of condoms

| | | Adjusted percentage who have ever used | | | | |
		15–19	20–24	25–39	40–49	50+
Côte d'Ivoire	Males	36	38	31	21	14
Côte d'Ivoire	Females	13	13	8	5	0
Lusaka	Males	59	61	42	20	7
Lusaka	Females	36	33	22	23	0

appreciably higher among the unmarried than the married. The multivariate analysis indicates that much of this association reflects the confounding influence of age, education and risk behaviour. For women, marital status emerges as a significant predictor for only one population. For men, there is a significant net effect in Manila and Rio de Janeiro but it proves to be of only minor substantive importance. Ever-use of condoms is higher among the small number of formerly married men, but there is no difference between the currently and never-married groups. Among Côte d'Ivoire males, there is a puzzling interaction between residence and marital status. In urban areas, use is lowest among the single population, but in rural areas there is a small difference in the opposite direction.

In contrast to marital status, the important influence of educational attainment on condom use is reaffirmed by logistic regression. This factor enters the model as a significant main effect in four male study populations and three of the female populations. Invariably, use is higher among the better educated. In some instances, the divergence, even after adjustment for all other regressions, is very large. For instance, 43 per cent of men with secondary schooling report use of the condom in Côte d'Ivoire compared to only 11 per cent of those with no schooling. The corresponding figures for men in Burundi and Lusaka are 30 and 45 for those with secondary schooling versus 11 and 22 for those with no schooling.

The final socio-demographic factor is rural–urban residence, which is applicable in only four of the six sites. Among Côte d'Ivoire females there is no significant net effect of residence on ever-use of condoms. In all the remaining seven study populations, there is a statistically significant main or interactive influence, with higher use in urban than in rural areas.

In contrast to the rather strong effects on condom use of the socio-demographic variables, other factors included in logistic regression do not emerge as predictors of condom use. Belief in sexual transmission of HIV has a significant net effect in only one study population and beliefs about the severity of AIDS in none of the six populations where this variable was measured. It is surprising to note that perceived personal risk of infection is also generally not related to ever-use of condoms. The main exception concerns men in Rio de Janeiro where use rises monotonically from 33 to 51 per cent as the sense of risk or personal vulnerability to AIDS increases. A similar effect is also found among the male population of Côte d'Ivoire but the gradient in use is much less pronounced, rising from 28 to only 36 per cent.

Finally, analysis of the link between exposure to information about AIDS and condom use yields slightly more positive results. In two of the three male populations where this relationship could be assessed, a large and statistically significant effect is found, in the expected direction. Among the female populations, however, only one significant result is apparent.

In conclusion, the major predictors of ever-use of condoms appear to be self-reported sexual behaviour plus the demographic factors of age, education and residence. The inability of the more psychological variables to predict condom use may reflect the fact that these variables refer to respondents' more recent experience with, and perception of, AIDS whereas the measure of condom use relates to a much longer reference period, predating the AIDS epidemic by several decades in the case of older age groups.

Before leaving the topic of condom use, it is appropriate to recall the results presented in the previous chapter on condom use within commercial sex encounters. Notwithstanding the strong link between non-marital sex and ever-use of condoms, it is apparent from Figure 4.18 that regular condom use for commercial sex was rather uncommon in 1989 or thereabouts. This result holds true not only among the African populations where ever-use of condoms is low and access is limited but also in other sites. Thus in Rio de Janeiro and Manila, about 80 per cent of men who reported recent contacts with sex workers had never used a condom on these occasions. In Thailand and Singapore, the levels of use are much higher but less than 30 per cent claimed to have used a condom on each occasion. Clearly, publicity for condom use in potentially high risk relationships is needed in all sites. There is, in addition, a pressing need for further intensive research on the determinants of condom use in these situations.

While use of condoms during contacts with sex workers is alarmingly low, it is lower still within marriage. The percentages of currently married men who reported use of condom on each occasion of intercourse with their wife or regular partner in the last four weeks are less than 10 per cent in nine of the twelve study populations where this information was gathered. Prevalence of regular condom use within marriage is slightly higher in Lusaka (11 per cent) and Lesotho (13 per cent). Only in Singapore, do a large minority (19 per cent) of couples rely on condoms.

Perceived Attributes of the Condom

This section presents the results of ten questions concerning attitudes towards condoms. The questions required respondents who had heard of the condom to express their agreement or disagreement with each of a number of statements about condoms. Respondents who did not have enough knowledge or confidence to give a definite response were free to express their lack of certainty by endorsing the *uncertain* or *don't know* response alternative. From the point of view of understanding the popular image or reputation of the condom in a population, these uncertain responses are as important as positive or negative replies. Psychologically, a high degree of uncertainty may be taken to indicate that the attribute in question is not yet a significant part of the image of the condom in the population concerned and, thus, is unlikely to play a major role in the acceptance and use of condoms. But, before this psychological interpretation is assumed, we need to examine the possibility that high levels of *uncertain/don't know* responses are not caused by difficulty in understanding the question or poor interviewer performance. In view of the different and relatively sophisticated format of these questions, it is essential to explore the possible impact of such artificial factors on the response patterns observed.

Exploratory analysis (not presented in detail here) reveals two interesting patterns. First, the proportion of respondents saying *don't know* varies considerably from one question to the other in a consistent manner in all research sites. Thus, certain questions are associated with high levels of uncertain responses in all research sites, while certain others have elicited a small number of uncertain responses across all sites. Second, items associated with low levels concern such long established and well known attributes as condoms' effectiveness as a contraceptive method, condoms' effectiveness against STDs, and condoms being appropriate for use with casual partners. Conversely, items which have elicited the largest amount of uncertainty in most sites deal with such culturally conditioned and subjectively defined characteristics as religious acceptability, ease of use and cost. These variations lend support to the assumption underlying the surveys that people will respond to the contents of individual items and in a logical and non-random manner. Further evidence in support of this interpretation and the validity of the findings is provided by the observation that, in all research sites, respondents who have not yet tried a condom and thus have no personal experience of various attributes are far more likely to give *uncertain/don't know* responses to all items than those who have already used a condom. This would not be the case if individuals had been answering the questions either in a random manner or just to appease the interviewer.

Table 5.8: Opinions on condoms: summary statistics for condom users and non-users

Statements	Males				Females			
	Mean Percentage Agreeing		Mean Percentage Uncertain/DK		Mean Percentage Agreeing		Mena Percentage Uncertain/DK	
	Condom Users	Non-users	Condom Users	Non-users	Condom Users	Non-users	Condom Users	Non-users
1. Condoms are good at preventing pregnancy	93	79	4	17	89	76	6	18
2. Condoms are good for preventing STDs	91	77	5	18	86	73	8	20
3. Condoms are easy to use	88	50	6	41	77	39	16	50
4. Condoms are too expensive	18	14	18	48	16	15	26	53
5. Condoms make sex less enjoyable	55	35	10	47	47	29	17	56
6. Condoms are appropriate for casual sex	78	65	8	22	70	58	13	28
7. Condoms are offensive to husbands/wives	39	37	13	33	33	36	14	35
8. Condoms are appropriate for spouse/reg. partner	38	24	14	31	47	27	15	33
9. Condoms are against my religion	18	21	20	32	18	21	22	35
10. Condoms may climb up into womb/stomach	32	24	15	46	27	23	21	48

In view of these considerations, the data have been analyzed separately for respondents who have only heard of condoms and those who have also used a condom once or more often. In the following presentation, the main emphasis will be on the proportion of respondents who agreed with specified statements. Results are presented in Table 5.8 in the form of overall mean results for all study populations.

Condoms can Prevent Pregnancy

In all research sites, the overwhelming majority of respondents agree that 'condoms, if used properly, can prevent unwanted pregnancy'. The proportion of the potential value of condoms as a means of contraception is particularly high among those who have ever used a condom. In fact, in 12 of the 14 populations, over 90 per cent of such respondents have agreed with this statement. Even among those who have not yet used a condom, over 70 per cent agreed with the effectiveness of condoms as a means of pregnancy control in all but one survey. The exception is Sri Lanka where a large majority (58 per cent) of respondents who have not used a condom expressed uncertainty regarding its effectiveness as a contraceptive. It may be of some interest to recall that the Sri Lanka sample has the lowest level of condom use and that, even among those who have used a condom, one quarter have expressed uncertainty regarding this attribute of the condom. There is little difference of opinion between men and women on this topic in all but one research site.

Condoms can Prevent Venereal Diseases

The overwhelming majority (70 to 95 per cent) of all respondents in all but one study population (Sri Lanka) also concurred that 'condoms can prevent venereal diseases' if used properly. Again, a higher proportion of respondents who have used a condom (81 to 98 per cent) than those who have only heard of it (66 to 94 per cent) agreed with this statement. Moreover, regardless of their experience with condoms, there is little difference between men and women on this point.

Condoms are Easy to Use

Regardless of whether they have used a condom or not, the majority of respondents in all research sites but Sri Lanka believed that 'condoms are easy to use'. The proportion endorsing this statement ranges from 72 to 95 per cent (median of 85.5 per cent) among ever-users and from 26 to 77 per cent (median of 43 per cent) among never-users.

In all research sites, larger proportions of men than women thought that condoms were easy to use. The differences are particularly noticeable in the Central African Republic (55 vs 35 per cent); Côte d'Ivoire (66 vs 43 per cent); Guinea Bissau (66 vs 40 per cent); Lesotho (74 vs 63 per cent); Tanzania (48 vs 38 per cent); Mauritius (70 vs 60 per cent); Manila (74 vs 44 per cent); Singapore (77 vs 51 per cent); Thailand (91 vs 76 per cent), and Rio de Janeiro (77 vs 56 per cent). These differences are primarily caused by the greater tendency of women than men to express uncertainty regarding the ease of use of condoms. This difference persists among users and non-users. As condoms are a male controlled prevention technology it is perhaps natural that men should have more firmly developed beliefs regarding their ease of use than women.

Condoms make Sex less Enjoyable

In 11 of the 14 research sites, the majority of respondents who have ever used a condom (48 to 71 per cent) concurred with the statement that 'Condoms make sex less enjoyable'. Only in Lesotho and Manila did the majority (49 and 57 per cent) disagree, and in Sri Lanka the majority (42 per cent) took an *uncertain* position. Among respondents with no history of condom use, the majority expressed uncertainty regarding this attribute of condoms in 10 of the 14 research sites. In all cases, however, there is a substantial minority who were uncertain. Regardless of their experience or lack of experience with condoms, more men than women endorsed the opinion that condoms make sex less enjoyable in all but two sites. The size of observed differences in favour of men exceeds 10 per cent in eight study populations.

Condoms are too Expensive to use Regularly

Except in Manila, the majority (39 to 86 per cent with a median of 63 per cent) of respondents who have ever used a condom disagreed that 'The price of condoms is too high to use regularly'. In Manila, the majority (68 per cent) were undecided. In the case of respondents who have not used a condom, the majority in ten research sites endorsed the uncertain response alternative and in five other sites the majority disagreed with the statement. In only seven instances (out of 30 possible comparisons), a substantial minority (over one-fifth) of respondents agreed with the statement regarding the cost of condoms being prohibitively high. Male/female differences with respect to this statement are mostly small and vary according to whether a condom has been used or not. Men who have used a condom outnumber their female counterparts in thinking that condoms are expensive by 10 percentage points or more in Côte d'Ivoire (42 vs 20 per cent); Burundi (21 vs 11 per cent); and Rio de Janeiro (31 vs 19 per cent).

Condoms are most Appropriate for Use with Non-regular Partners

There is a high degree of consensus among respondents from different sites that 'condoms are most appropriate for use with non-regular partners'. Disregarding the Sri Lanka sample, the proportion of respondents agreeing with this statement ranges from 58 per cent to 94 per cent (with a median of 78 per cent) among those who have used a condom and from 51 per cent to 89 per cent (median being 62 per cent) among those who have only heard of condoms. Thus between 58 per cent and 91 per cent (median of 68 per cent) of all respondents from 13 different sites (excluding Sri Lanka) agreed that condoms are most appropriate for use outside of stable partnerships. In Sri Lanka, 50 per cent of ever-users and 77 per cent of never-users expressed uncertainty regarding this attribute of the condom. More men than women agreed with this statement in all research sites. The sex difference in favour of men is particularly noteworthy in Côte d'Ivoire (82 vs 66 per cent); Guinea Bissau (76 vs 64 per cent); Mauritius (76 vs 59 per cent); Manila (78 vs 61 per cent); and Singapore (64 vs 52 per cent).

Condoms are most Appropriate for Use with Spouse/Regular Partner

There is an interesting divide in opinion between research sites in the perceived appropriateness of condom use within marriage. In four sites (Lesotho, Singapore, Mauritius, and Lusaka) the large majority (57 to 76 per cent) of respondents who have ever used a condom concurred with the statement that 'condoms are most appropriate for use with spouse/regular partner'. In seven other sites (Central African Republic, Côte d'Ivoire, Guinea Bissau, Burundi, Tanzania, Thailand and Rio de Janeiro) the majority (48 to 80 per cent) disagreed with this position. In the two remaining populations (Sri Lanka and Manila), the majority expressed uncertainty. Among respondents who have not yet used a condom, the majority endorsed the uncertain response alternative in four research sites (Tanzania, Manila, Singapore, and Sri Lanka).

In nine of the 14 study populations, more women than men agreed that condoms are appropriate for use with spouse/regular partner. In the whole sample, however, the observed male/female differences are mostly small (less than 10 per cent) and thus there appears to be no systematic divergence between opinions of men and women. However, differences become larger among the condom experienced sub-sample where women outnumber men by ten percentage points or more in terms of believing that condoms are appropriate for use with regular partners in the following surveys: Togo (56 vs 30 per cent); Burundi (48 vs 34 per cent); Lusaka (64 vs 52 per cent); Mauritius (74 vs 61 per cent); Thailand (42 vs 27 per cent); and Rio de Janeiro (38 vs 12 per cent).

Condoms are Offensive to Spouse/Regular Partner

There is an interesting diversity of opinion among respondents from different sites regarding the perceived offensiveness of condoms to spouses/regular partners. Of the whole samples surveyed, more respondents agreed than disagreed with the statement in eight of the 14 research sites. Interestingly, all but one of these are in sub-Saharan Africa. On the other hand, of the six populations where more respondents disagreed with this statement, only one is African (Burundi).

In only two surveys (Guinea Bissau, 52 per cent, and Thailand, 55 per cent), a small absolute majority of all respondents agreed that 'condoms are offensive to husbands/wives/regular sex partners' and only in three sites (Mauritius, 51 per cent; Manila, 53 per cent; and Rio de Janeiro, 54 per cent) a clear majority of all respondents disagreed with this statement. A similarly small majority of respondents who have ever used a condom endorsed this statement in the Central African Republic (55 per cent), Guinea Bissau (50 per cent), and Tanzania (59 per cent). Among respondents who know of the condom but have not yet tried it, an overall majority agreed with this statement in Guinea Bissau (52 per cent) and Thailand (58 per cent) only. Leaving aside the uncertain respondents (who account for 4 to 44 per cent of condom users and 8 to 81 per cent of non-users in different sites), it would appear that, in over half of the sites (that is, in 8 out of 14), people are more likely to agree that condoms are offensive to spouse/regular partner than to disagree. In six other sites, however, a clear majority of respondents disagreed with this statement. Four of the latter sites are outside continental Africa and three of them (Mauritius, Singapore, and Rio de Janeiro) have very high levels of condom use.

A larger proportion of men than women respondents in general agreed with this statement in eight of the 14 sites. Among respondents who have already used the condom, larger proportions of men than women thought condoms were offensive in 11 cases. Togo is the only major exception to this generalization.

Condoms may Climb up into the Womb/Stomach

This mistaken fear is believed to be commonly held in many developing countries. According to the findings of the WHO/GPA surveys, a considerable minority (5 to 49 per cent, with a median of about 27 per cent) of all respondents thought that 'condoms can climb up into the womb or stomach', but only in Togo does the proportion of respondents concurring with this position approach 50 per cent. On the other hand, in only five research sites did a majority of respondents disagree with this statement. Three of these are outside Africa. Even among respondents who have already used a condom, relatively large proportions particularly in Africa (ranging from 8 to 61 per cent) agree that condoms can climb into the womb or stomach.

Many people endorsing this statement may be led to do so by equating it with the idea of condom breakage and slipping off the penis. This is the interpretation clearly implied in the Côte d'Ivoire and Thai versions of the questionnaire. In any case, it is encouraging to note that in nine of the 11 surveys with the necessary data, a large majority of respondents who have ever used a condom disagreed with this statement. Only in Côte d'Ivoire and Togo, did large proportions (46 per cent and 61 per cent) of respondents with some experience of condom use concur with the statement. Among respondents with no experience of condom use, the majority of respondents in Thailand (51 per cent) and Rio de Janeiro (60 per cent) disagreed with the statement, while the majority in Togo (46 per cent) agreed with it. In the remaining eight research sites the majority of never-user respondents expressed uncertainty.

Opinions of men and women are similar. In only four countries (Côte d'Ivoire, Guinea Bissau, Burundi and Kenya) did the proportion of men and women agreeing with this statement differ by 10 percentage points or more. In all these cases, a smaller proportion of women than men concurred with the statement that condoms may climb up into the womb or stomach.

Condoms are Against my Religion

In nine of the 15 study populations, a large majority of all respondents disagreed with the statement that 'Condom use is against my religion'. Disagreement is higher among respondents who have ever used a condom. Only in Tanzania, did a small majority (40 per cent) of such respondents agree with the statement and only in Manila did the majority (64 per cent) of such respondents take an uncertain position regarding the relationship of condoms and religion. Among respondents with no experience of condom use, too, the majority disagreed that condom use is against their religion in nine of 15 research sites. Kenya is an exception where a substantial proportion (38 per cent) of the never-users agreed that condom is against their religion. In the remaining five research sites they expressed uncertainty. There is little variation by sex of respondent with regard to this belief in all research sites but one.

Condoms and HIV Prevention

In eight research sites where the KABP interview schedule was used, respondents who had heard of the condom and who had also indicated an awareness of AIDS in response to earlier questions, were asked if they thought that condoms could prevent AIDS. Results are summarized in Figure 5.4. With the exception of Guinea Bissau, it would appear that, among respondents with some knowledge of AIDS and the condom, less than half knew that condoms can prevent AIDS. The proportion of respondents with such knowledge was particularly low in Thailand (11 per cent) and Burundi (24 per cent). In all sites, fewer women than men knew of this attitude of the condom. The proportion of respondents who knew that condoms can prevent AIDS increases consistently and considerably by level of education, place of residence, and exposure to mass media of communication in all eight research sites. People who have ever used a condom were much more likely to be aware of this property of the condom.

These findings contrast sharply with the results of the attitude item regarding the ability of condoms to prevent venereal diseases discussed above.

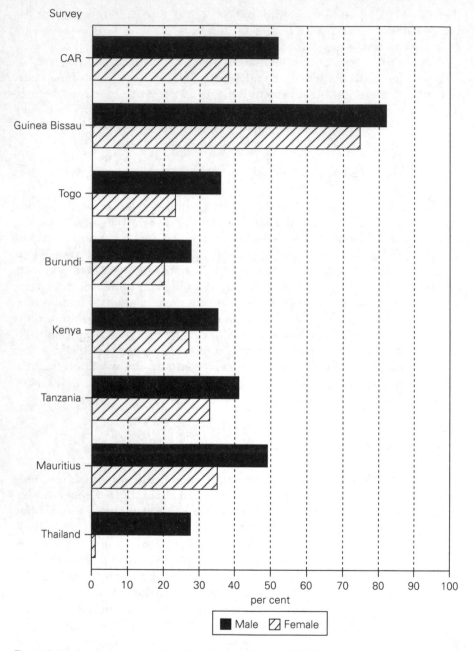

Survey

Figure 5.4:   *Among males and females who have heard of AIDS and of condoms, the percentage who know that condoms can prevent HIV*

The differences may be partly due to the rather indirect way in which the question regarding the ability of the condom to prevent AIDS was worded. Respondents who had mentioned one or more contraceptives (including condoms) were asked if they knew that any of these could be used to prevent AIDS. It is also likely that, in view of their longer experience with traditional STDs, respondents have learned about the ability of condoms to prevent them but this knowledge has not yet been generalized to HIV/AIDS. The practical conclusion for AIDS education campaigns may be that they should promote condoms explicitly for HIV/AIDS prevention rather than STD control or family planning.

Conclusions and Implications

Several important points have emerged from the analysis. First, populations represented by these WHO/GPA surveys differ considerably in terms of familiarity with the condom. With few exceptions, populations in sub-Saharan Africa are less likely than populations elsewhere to have heard of the condom. Second, inter-country variations with regard to ever having used a condom are even more remarkable. Relatively small proportions of all respondents report personal use of a condom in most sites. Although the levels of condom use rise to varying extents when the sexually experienced segment of the population is considered, the absolute figures observed in most sites are far from impressive in the era of AIDS. Again with some exceptions, the sub-Saharan African populations included in this analysis manifested much lower levels of condom use than populations elsewhere. In view of the urgency of the AIDS situation in Africa and its potential for becoming urgent in Asian and central and southern American societies in the near future, the findings of these surveys point to the need for further and more vigorous condom promotion campaigns.

The general findings as well as regional variations in condom awareness and use revealed by the WHO/GPA surveys are consistent with findings of earlier data collected by the World Fertility Surveys, Demographic and Health Surveys and other Contraceptive Prevalence/Family Planning Surveys regarding the discouragingly low levels of condom awareness and utilization in most developing countries, particularly those in sub-Saharan Africa. Clearly, the emphasis of most family planning programmes in sub-Saharan Africa (Caldwell and Caldwell, 1986; Frank, 1987) has hardly prepared people either to deal with the problem of traditional STDs – and the high rates of infertility and other adverse health outcomes often associated with them – or to cope with the challenge of the HIV pandemic.

Consistent intra-country variations of condom awareness and use levels by such characteristics as sex, residence, media exposure and level of education are also in line with results of earlier contraceptive prevalence surveys. These findings underline the importance of general socio-economic development for the adoption of new attitudes and instruments of family planning and reproductive health. Nevertheless, the importance of deliberate strategies for promoting condoms as a means of contraception or STD control, particularly among women, cannot be overemphasized.

Lack of knowledge of condoms can be overcome relatively easily by extensive publicity. Experience with family planning programmes over the last 30 years has demonstrated beyond doubt that awareness of major methods of contraception can be raised to very high levels within a short period of time, provided that the political will exists to make use of radio, television, posters and other methods of communication. The next logical step in condom promotion is to increase access, for unless individuals can obtain supplies from a nearby source, actual use of condoms is bound to be limited. Ideally condom access should be assessed objectively by means of community enquiries. In the WHO/GPA surveys, a different, and less satisfactory, approach was used, whereby persons aware of condoms were asked whether they knew a supply source and, if so, how long it would take to visit that place. The majority of those aware of condoms were also knowledgable about potential supply sources; nevertheless, in a number of populations, about one in five of respondents was unaware of any source and in two sites this proportion exceeds 30 per cent. Clearly, awareness of the method does not necessarily imply awareness of a source. Moreover, in two West African surveys, large proportions of respondents who claimed to know a source were unable to estimate travelling time to that source, implying very superficial acquaintance with potential sources.

Effective access to condoms may be defined in the following terms. A person must have heard of condoms, must be aware of a supply source and must live (or work) within 30 minutes of it. The application of this criterion of access reveals the huge challenge for condom promotion, particularly in Africa. Among the six African surveys for which relevant data are available, the percentage of all men classified as possessing effective access to condoms ranges from 15 to 38 per cent. For women, these figures are even lower. It is thus hardly surprising that use of condoms is so low.

While physical access is one important determinant of use, financial access may be an equally powerful influence. No attempt in these surveys was made to estimate the actual cost, but respondents were asked whether they thought that the price of condoms was too high for regular use. Perhaps surprisingly, price did not emerge as a commonly perceived constraint on use. Averaging across all surveys, only about 15 per cent of men and women conceded that high cost prevented regular use. However, these opinions are no substitute for experimental evidence on the price elasticity of condom use.

Further possible barriers to condom use were explored by assessing the popular image of condoms on a number of attributes. Overall, the general impression is rather favourable. Large majorities considered that condoms were effective for pregnancy and STD prevention and were easy to use.

Similarly, few men or women implied that their use would be contrary to religious beliefs. More substantial minorities, particularly among men, expressed concern about health risks of condom use for women. Such misconceptions that condoms can enter the womb or stomach clearly need to be dispelled in some populations. The most obvious potential objection to condom use is that sexual enjoyment is reduced. About half of all men and women who had used condoms agreed that this was so, as did about one-third of non-users. This negative attribute of condoms has been recognized for many years and has been addressed by exotic brand names, and other marketing devices.

At the outset of this chapter, the historical association of condoms with illicit sex was mentioned. This association persists strongly in some settings. Respondents were much more likely to consider condoms appropriate for non-marital sexual contacts than within a regular partnership; averaged across all surveys, nearly 40 per cent of respondents agreed that condom use would be offensive to a spouse or regular partner. The data on this topic suggest that women are somewhat less likely to reject condom use within marriage than men, a potentially important point that could be exploited in promotion campaigns.

The implications of this finding for HIV prevention are not straightforward. One obvious priority is to encourage condom use for protection in non-marital sexual encounters, particularly of a commercial or fleeting nature. But publicity to reinforce this behaviour may be counterproductive in terms of risk reduction within stable partnerships. Once HIV has spread into the general heterosexual population, this issue becomes of increasing concern and too close an identification of condoms with extra-marital contacts damages the likelihood that individuals, fearful of infection by their regular partner, will insist upon condom use.

The evidence from these surveys shows a strong link between non-marital sex and condom use. Typically those who report extra-marital sex within the last 12 months were twice as likely to have tried condoms than those reporting no sex outside marriage. However as Figure 4.18 in Chapter 4 indicates, regular condom use, even in commercial sex encounters, is the exception rather than the rule in all study populations. In seven of the ten surveys with relevant data, more than half of all men reporting commercial sex in the last 12 months had never used a condom on these occasions; and the proportion who had used condoms on all occasions were typically 20 per cent or less. Clearly an immediate priority is to increase condom use in such relationships. One way to do so is to make people aware that HIV transmission can be greatly reduced, if not totally eliminated, by the proper use of latex condoms. This belief is not yet well established in the populations covered by the WHO/GPA surveys. Among respondents with some awareness of HIV/AIDS and condoms, less than half knew that condoms are effective against transmission of HIV. Moreover, as will be shown in Chapter 6, men who did use condoms for commercial sex are just as likely to feel at risk of

HIV infection as those who did not use condoms. The difficult challenge ahead is to raise drastically levels of condom use in potentially high risk ephemeral sexual contacts, without diminishing the chance that they will be used, when appropriate, in more regular relationships.

Chapter 6

Risk Perception and Behavioural Change

John Cleland

Introduction

It has become a cliché to state that behavioural change is the only way of arresting the HIV pandemic, until such time that an effective vaccine or cure is discovered. As for many clichés, mindless repetition should not be allowed to undermine its validity. Indeed, behavioural modification is probably even more important than is implied above. There is no guarantee that a biomedical solution will be found; even if one is found, it remains uncertain whether it can be applied with sufficient thoroughness to act as a panacea. The history of other sexually transmitted diseases should serve as a warning in this regard. Though effective cures for many of them have existed for decades, they still remain a major public health problem, with a high incidence particularly in Africa (e.g. Schulz, Cates and O'Mara, 1987).

Behavioural change is the most important topic to be addressed in this chapter. It is also the most difficult to measure and interpret using data from single-round surveys. As we shall see, the results are both encouraging but, at the same time, should not be interpreted literally. Substantial proportions of men and women in many of the surveys say that they have already changed their behaviour in response to the threat of AIDS. Moreover, the main changes mentioned are potentially effective ways of reducing the risk of HIV transmission. But these reports are undoubtedly exaggerated. There is no evidence to corroborate behavioural change on the massive scale suggested by the survey findings. It appears probable that many respondents are merely giving a verbal acquiescence to the desirability or need for change. Yet, even this cautious interpretation provides grounds for optimism. The prognosis for the further spread of HIV would be much more gloomy had the majority of individuals denied any personal need to modify their behaviour.

The material on the behavioural response to AIDS comes towards the end of the chapter. The earlier sections concern the perceived general threat of AIDS to communities or countries and the extent to which individuals see themselves to be at risk of infection. This information complements the findings in Chapter 3 on awareness of AIDS, beliefs about transmission and its perceived severity. In rationalistic models of human behaviour, all these factors are expected to influence the probability of adaptive behaviour modification.

No explicit or implicit assumption should be made that rational models of human behaviour offer complete or satisfying understanding of change. Indeed the record of psychological models, associated with the work of Becker, Ajzen, Fishbein and others, in predicting behavioural outcomes is mixed. Furthermore, many factors, not covered in WHO/GPA surveys, are likely to influence behaviours, not least attitudes towards the behaviours that require modification, external impediments to change and social pressures. Nevertheless, the factors discussed in the first part of the chapter, together with those covered in Chapter 3, may be considered as necessary, if not sufficient, preconditions for change. In order for an appropriate behavioural response to a disease to occur, an individual must be aware of it, be knowledgable of ways to reduce risk of infection, acknowledge its health-threatening nature, feel some sense of personal vulnerability to it and finally feel able to reduce risk by behaviour. The WHO/GPA surveys can illuminate all these preconditions, in a manner that is highly relevant to prevention strategies.

Perceptions of the General Threat of AIDS

In order to assess respondents' perceptions of HIV/AIDS in relation to other health issues, two open-ended questions were posed in KABP surveys: *What do you think are the most serious diseases or health problems facing the world today?* and *What do you think are the most serious diseases or health problems facing your country today?* Answers to both questions were recorded verbatim, but they were coded solely in terms of whether or not AIDS was mentioned. It should be stressed that these questions preceded any explicit items on HIV/AIDS. Indeed, respondents had not even been asked whether they had heard of the disease. Because of this early location in the questionnaire, answers should not have been conditioned by the central focus of the interview. It remains possible, nevertheless, that news of the subject matter of the enquiry spread within selected sample areas. To the extent that such diffusion occurred, respondents were forewarned of the nature of the survey and their answers may have been biased towards mention of AIDS.

As the PR questionnaire did not include the relevant questions, results, shown in Figure 6.1, are confined to a sub-set of eight surveys. Their most remarkable feature is the high proportion of respondents who mentioned AIDS as one of the most serious diseases facing the world. In all but one survey, over half cited AIDS, and the proportion rises to about 70 per cent or more in the four east and southern African surveys. The single main exception is Togo, where only one-quarter of all respondents cited AIDS as a serious global disease. At this juncture, it should be recalled that the Togo survey, like several others, was conducted in 1989 at the very early stages of

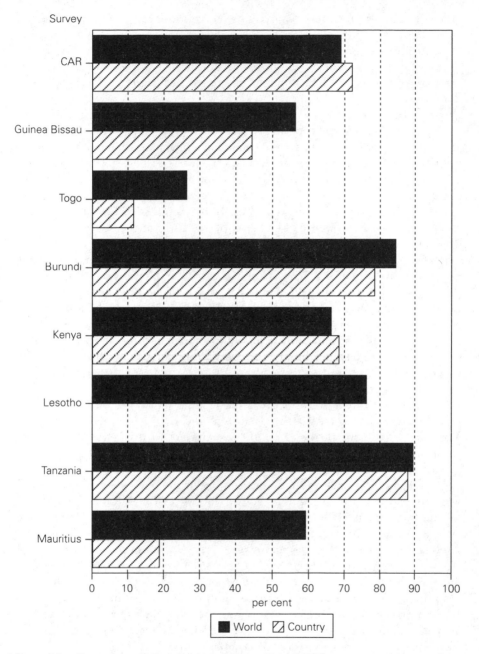

Figure 6.1: Percentage of all respondents who mentioned AIDS spontaneously as one of the most serious diseases (a) facing the world; (b) facing the country/community

HIV-control and prevention campaigns. Perceptions may well have changed since that time. Nevertheless, it is reasonable to suggest, that in the late 1980s, Togo lagged behind the other countries represented in Figure 6.1 in terms of recognition of the global seriousness of the pandemic. The low level of awareness of AIDS in Togo, discussed in Chapter 3, reinforces this diagnosis.

Togo also proves to be an exception in another regard. In most surveys, there was little difference between the proportions mentioning AIDS as a *global* health problem and as a *national* health problem. In Togo, this correspondence was not found: respondents were twice as likely to mention AIDS as a world problem than as a national problem (26 versus 12 per cent). An even more clear-cut distinction may be observed in Mauritius, where the corresponding proportions were 59 and 19 per cent. As very few HIV positive cases had been identified in Mauritius by the time of the survey, this large difference is readily understandable.

How many of those persons who had heard of AIDS spontaneously mentioned it as one of the most serious diseases? The answer is given by a comparison of Figure 6.1 with Table 3.1, which shows the level of awareness of AIDS. The results for the Central African Republic and Guinea Bissau are typical of most surveys. In the former survey, 83 per cent were aware of AIDS and 72 per cent (equivalent to nearly 90 per cent of those aware) cited it as one of the most serious global health problems. In Guinea Bissau, the gap is wider: yet 75 per cent of those aware of AIDS spontaneously mentioned it as a serious health problem. This pattern holds true for most of the other surveys: among those aware of the disease, large majorities rank it highly in terms of seriousness, both at international and national levels. Once again, Togo and Mauritius prove to be the exceptions to this generalization. In these surveys, the number of respondents who had heard of AIDS was much greater than the number considering it as a serious problem.

A second approach to the measurement of the perceived threat of AIDS was used in the KABP instrument. At the start of section 4, following a battery of questions about AIDS knowledge and sources of information, respondents were asked the following two questions: *How much of a threat do you think AIDS is to the health of your local community **now**?* and *How about the next few years? Is AIDS going to be a serious threat to the health of this community?* The permissible answers *(no threat at all; some threat; serious threat)* were read out to each respondent. Minor variations to these questions occurred in specific surveys. In some instances, the word *country* was used instead of *community*; and in Kenya, the answer categories were expanded. However, these variations do not represent a serious erosion of comparability.

Results are summarized in Figure 6.2, in terms of the percentage of respondents answering that AIDS is (or will be) a serious health threat. Of particular note is the pattern of response in Mauritius, Manila and Singapore. All three areas had very low levels of HIV infection at the time of their respective surveys. Yet appreciable proportions, ranging from nearly 30 per

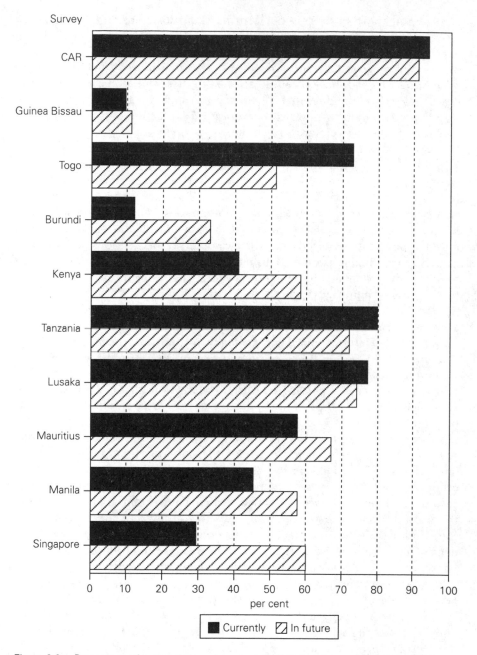

Figure 6.2: Percentage of respondents who perceive AIDS threat as serious: (a) currently; (b) in the future (restricted to those aware of AIDS)

cent in Singapore to over 50 per cent in Mauritius, considered AIDS to be a serious threat. Furthermore, the threat of AIDS was thought to be increasing; around 60 per cent of all respondents aware of AIDS considered that the disease will represent a serious health threat in the future. While the context of the interview may have coloured answers to these questions, the results are nevertheless encouraging; there is no support here for the frequent suggestion that populations with very low levels of HIV infection dismiss the general threat of AIDS as irrelevant or remote.

The results from the African surveys vary widely. In the Central African Republic, Togo, Tanzania and Lusaka, over 70 per cent of respondents (amongst those aware of AIDS) recognize AIDS as a serious threat to the health of their communities. The results for Togo are rather unexpected in view of the small proportion who had spontaneously mentioned AIDS as one of the most serious global or national diseases. In all four surveys, slightly fewer respondents reported that AIDS was likely to be a serious health threat in the future, than at present. This pattern contrasts strongly with the results for Mauritius, Manila, and Singapore, where the future threat was perceived to be greater than that currently pertaining.

In the Kenyan survey, 40 per cent of respondents considered AIDS to be a current threat but, in contrast to respondents in the Central African Republic, Togo, Tanzania and Lusaka, a higher proportion (nearly 60 per cent) thought that AIDS would be a serious threat in the future. Response in the remaining two surveys – Guinea Bissau and Burundi – are very different. Only about 10 per cent considered AIDS to be a serious threat. This proportion rises in Burundi to 30 per cent in answer to the question about the future, but not in Guinea Bissau. These results are puzzling because spontaneous answers to the earlier questions (see Figure 6.1) offered no suggestion that AIDS might be perceived to be a relatively unimportant issue in these two countries. In Guinea Bissau, a plausible explanation for the apparent discrepancy lies in the very high proportions who were unable to give a definite response; 37 per cent were classified as being uncertain about the current threat of AIDS and this proportion rises to 51 per cent in relation to the future threat. In Burundi, *don't know* responses comprise a little over 10 per cent of all answers and thus there is no obvious resolution of the discrepancy between the results of the earlier and the later questions.

To sum up, answers to these questions suggest that there is a willingness among adults to recognize the general threat and seriousness of AIDS. Separate analyses (not reported on here) indicate men and women hold similar beliefs in this regard. In the majority of surveys, AIDS is mentioned spontaneously by over half of all respondents as one of the most serious health problems facing the world and the country. Answers to more focused questions provide similar indications. In seven of the ten surveys, over 40 per cent of respondents rated AIDS as a *serious threat* rather than *some threat* or *no threat at all.* In some of the African surveys, however, there is little awareness that the problem may worsen in the future. By contrast, the populations of

Manila, Singapore and Mauritius see a greater threat in the future than at present.

Perceived Personal Risk of Infection by HIV/AIDS

Following the questions about the threat of AIDS to the community, respondents were asked the following much more personal question: *What are the chances that you yourself might catch AIDS? Would you say: not likely at all, very small chance, moderate chance, good chance, do not know?*

As mentioned earlier, the concept of personal risk, or vulnerability, is central to many theories of behavioural change. Indeed in some theories, the feeling of personal risk is held to be a precondition for adaptive change. Because of this centrality, the item was included in both KABP and PR instruments. However, a number of survey-specific adaptations were made to the wording of the question. The most common was to collapse the permissible answers into four instead of five. Respondents were asked to classify themselves as having a small, intermediate or high risk of contracting HIV/AIDS, with an additional option of uncertainty (i.e. don't know). The precise terms used to describe these options varied. For instance, Singaporean respondents had to choose between *not likely at all, somewhat likely* and *very likely*, and Mauritians between *no risk, small risk, big risk*. Surveys also varied in handling of the *don't know* or uncertain responses. In Thailand, this type of answer was not permitted and, in the Central African Republic, only 0.1 per cent was classified as responding this way. In several other surveys, however, between one-quarter and one-third of all answers were coded as uncertain. These divergencies undoubtedly complicate the cross-cultural comparability of responses, and the problem is further exacerbated by the fact that these gradations of risk had to be conveyed, in many instances, by means of local languages and dialects. Interpretative caution is therefore essential.

The key results are shown in Figure 6.3. We have chosen a display that emphasizes the distinction between the relatively unambiguous response *not likely* (to the left of the central line) and the other responses that denote recognition of some personal risk or uncertainty. For surveys that adhered to the standard question, the responses of *moderate chance* and *good chance* have been combined to form a single high risk group.

In terms of the percentage of respondents who saw themselves at little or no risk of infection, the fifteen surveyed populations fell into two groups. The first comprises those where over 50 per cent expressed no personal risk. In here fall all the Asian populations, Mauritius and Lusaka. In the other group are all the remaining African countries and Rio de Janeiro, where the proportions denying personal risk range from 20 to about 40 per cent.

These two broad groupings correspond broadly to the spread of the pandemic within specific countries at the time of their respective surveys. For instance Mauritius, Manila, Singapore and Sri Lanka had reported very few

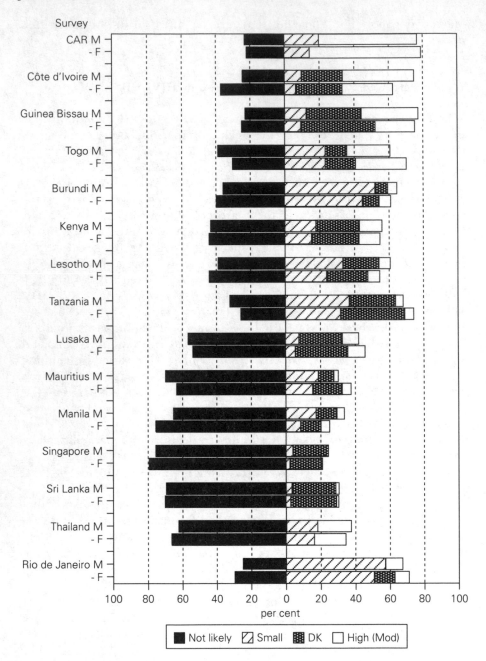

Figure 6.3: Per cent distribution of male (M) and (F) respondents according to perceived personal risk of AIDS (restricted to those aware of AIDS)

HIV infections or cases of AIDS at the time, and thus it is not surprising that large proportions of the populations surveyed felt themselves to be at low risk. Conversely, in most of the African countries represented here, the disease had penetrated at least the urban population by the late 1980s; hence, lower proportions denying risk are to be expected in these settings. The two main exceptions to this link between the spread of HIV within countries and perceptions of personal risk are Lusaka and Thailand. In both cases the proportions of men and women saying that they were at little or no risk are much higher than in other countries with similar levels of HIV infection. There are a number of possible explanations, including the nature and intensity of public information campaigns in Lusaka and Thailand and patterns of risk behaviour among these populations.

We turn now to consider the other extreme response: perception of a moderate or high risk. The most striking feature is the very high proportions considering themselves to be at appreciable risk among the four francophone countries of central and west Africa (Table 6.1 and Figure 6.3). Over one in four of all respondents (among those aware of AIDS) in the Central African Republic, Côte d'Ivoire, Guinea Bissau and Togo classified themselves in this manner. By contrast, the corresponding proportions for the east and southern African countries range from 5 to 13 per cent. As expected, few men or women see themselves to be at significant risk in Mauritius, Manila, or Singapore. The proportion is higher in Rio de Janeiro (9 per cent) and higher still in Thailand (19 per cent). The result for Thailand is of special interest, because of the high proportions denying risk. It appears that risk perceptions are more polarized in this country than elsewhere. The same point can be made in relation to Lusaka.

It is evident from both Figure 6.3 and Table 6.1 that risk perceptions vary little between men and women. Only two exceptions should be noted. In Côte d'Ivoire and Guinea Bissau, men are more likely than women to report themselves at risk.

How do feelings of personal susceptibility to AIDS relate to reported risk behaviour? The answer to this question is sought in Figure 6.4. As few women in most surveys reported risk behaviours, the analysis is confined to men. Figure 6.4 shows the risk perceptions of the following four behavioural groups:

- High risk: commercial sex reported in last 12 months
- Medium risk: no commercial sex reported but sexual contacts outside regular partnerships reported in the last 12 months
- Low risk: no sex outside regular partnerships reported in the last 12 months
- No risk: no sexual contacts at all reported in the last 12 months

These categories represent only one way of ranking risk behaviour. Moreover, the typology is an oversimplified representation of exposure to the risk of sexual transmission of HIV because it does not take account of

Table 6.1: Among respondents aware of AIDS, the percentage who report that they are at moderate or high risk of HIV infection

Survey	Men	Women	All
Central African Republic	57	64	60
Côte d'Ivoire	43	29	37
Guinea Bissau	34	24	30
Togo	26	20	27
Burundi	6	6	6
Kenya	14	13	13
Lesotho	8	8	8
Tanzania	5	6	5
Lusaka	10	10	10
Mauritius	3	4	3
Manila	5	5	5
Singapore	1	0	0
Sri Lanka	2	2	2
Thailand	20	18	19
Rio de Janeiro	10	8	9

condom use, number of partners, or nature of partners beyond the crude commercial/non-commercial distinction. Nevertheless, it suffices to establish the nature and approximate magnitude of the relationship between reported sexual behaviour and perception of personal risk. The immediate and dominant impression from Figure 6.4 is that this link is much weaker than might be expected on assumptions that the main routes of HIV transmission are known; feelings of susceptibility are entirely rational; and individuals have reported accurately their sexual behaviour in the last 12 months. In nearly half of the surveys (Central African Republic, Guinea Bissau, Mauritius, Manila, Singapore, and Sri Lanka) there is no clear-cut relationship between reported risk behaviour and risk perception. In a further two surveys (Côte d'Ivoire, Burundi), the relationship is not pronounced. This leaves Kenya, Lesotho, Tanzania, Lusaka, Thailand and Rio de Janeiro. In these surveys, the expected link emerges: the greater the reported risk behaviour, the higher is the proportion of men who perceive themselves to be vulnerable to infection. Among this latter group of surveys the relationship is monotonic. Men who report commercial sex are most likely to feel at risk of contracting HIV, followed sequentially by those who have had sex outside of regular partnerships, those who report sex within regular partnerships only, and finally those who report no sexual relationships at all in the preceding twelve months.

The pattern of results for the four francophone countries of central and west Africa is again particularly puzzling. Not only is the overall proportion stating themselves to be at appreciable risk very large, but, even among men who report no sex in the last 12 months, these proportions remain high (Central African Republic, 52; Côte d'Ivoire, 27; Guinea Bissau, 27; Togo, 27). The corresponding figure for all other surveys is below 15 per cent. It is possible that the pattern arises from misunderstanding of questions or gross misreporting of sexual risk behaviour. Alternatively, this contrast may

Survey/Risk behaviour

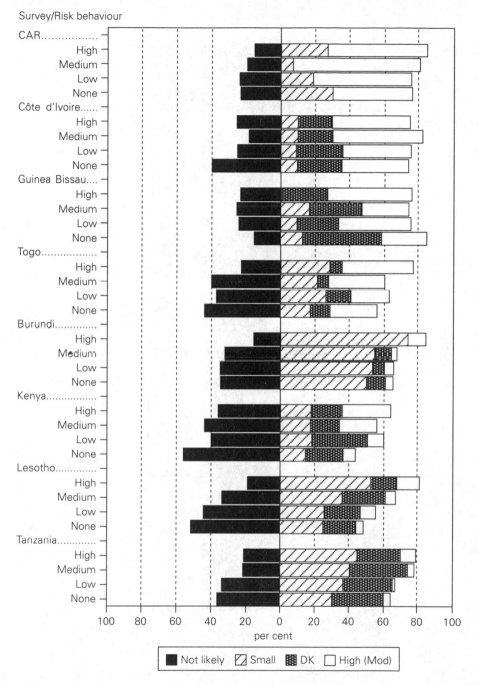

Figure 6.4: Per cent distribution of male respondents according to perceived personal risk of AIDS by reported risk behaviour in the last 12 months

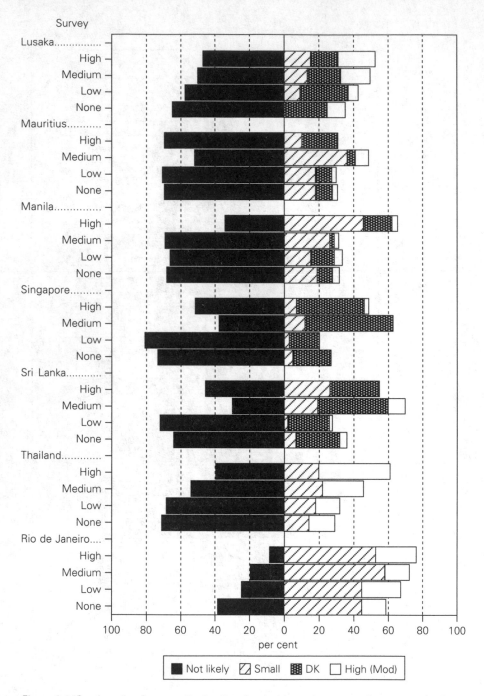

Figure 6.4 (Continued):   Per cent distribution of male respondents according to perceived
personal risk of AIDS by reported risk behaviour in the last 12 months

Table 6.2: Among men who reported commercial sex in last 12 months, the percentage reporting personal risk of AIDS, by whether or not condoms were used regularly

	Percentage	N
Central African Republic		
Used	28*	34
Not used	13	146
Côte d'Ivoire		
Used	41	22
Not used	28	221
Guinea Bissau		
Used	21	24
Not used	23	35
Tanzania		
Used	19	58
Not used	18	647
Lusaka		
Used	59	27
Not used	47	86
Singapore		
Used	52	21
Not used	51	53
Thailand		
Used	52*	89
Not used	38	189

* Statistically significant difference (p < 0.05)

have a cognitive or cultural basis; beliefs in casual, or even magical transmission of AIDS, may be more common in central and west Africa than elsewhere, thus accounting for a very widespread, diffuse sense of vulnerability, that appears to have no rational basis in behaviour. The evidence presented in Chapter 3 provides some support for this view. Ability to distinguish accurately between sexual and casual transmission tends to be lower in west and central than in east and southern Africa; and beliefs in transmission through insect bites are appreciably higher (Table 3.3).

The classification of risk behaviour in Figure 6.4 takes no account of condom use. However, respondents who reported commercial sex in the last 12 months were asked about use of condoms in these encounters. These data allow us to assess whether or not regular use of condoms with sex workers influences perceptions of risk. Table 6.2 compares the perceived personal risk of men who regularly used condoms for commercial sex with those of men who occasionally or never used condoms. The comparison can only be performed for a sub-set of surveys with sufficient numbers of men reporting condom use. Even after this selection, it is apparent from Table 6.2 that very small minorities of men in most surveys reported regular use of condoms. Nor is there a uniform difference in risk perception between them and non-users or irregular users of condoms across all seven surveys represented in

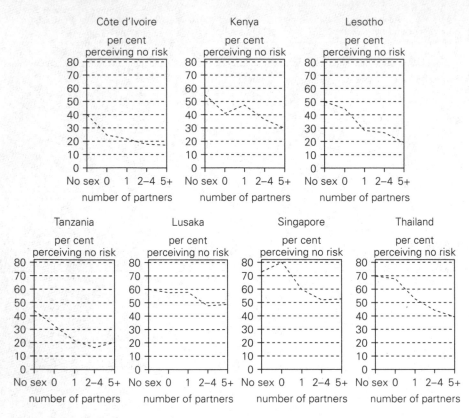

Figure 6.5: Percentage of men reporting no personal risk of AIDS, by number of reported non-regular/commercial partners in the last 12 months

the Table. In the Central African Republic, Guinea Bissau, Côte d'Ivoire and Thailand, regular users of condoms express less personal vulnerability to HIV infection than others. In the other three surveys, the relationship is weak. The difference is statistically significant for only two of the seven surveys. It is also of concern to note that many irregular or non-users of condoms feel themselves to be at no risk of HIV infection. Because of strict health surveillance of sex workers in Singapore, this feeling of low risk may have some justification. But in the other settings, the public health implications are serious.

Epidemiological studies indicate that one of the most consistent behavioural predictors of STD or HIV infection is the number of sexual partners, or rate of partner change. As noted earlier, one of the weaknesses of the risk behaviour classification used in Figure 6.4 is that it takes no explicit account of this dimension. This defect is remedied in Figure 6.5, which shows the proportion of men who perceive themselves to be at no risk of HIV/AIDS, classified by number of non-regular or commercial partners in the last 12

Table 6.3: Socio-demographic differentials in proportions of respondents who consider themselves at moderate or high risk of contracting AIDS

Survey	Age less than 25 vs. 25–49 (=1.00)	Never-married vs. currently married (=1.00)	Secondary+ School vs. Primary or no school (=1.00)	Urban vs. Rural (=1.00)
CAR	.99	.97	1.07	1.08
Côte d'Ivoire	1.00	1.01	1.58	1.42
Guinea Bissau	.99	1.06	1.53	.95
Togo	.81	.83	1.03	1.05
Burundi	.89	.91	1.23	1.19
Kenya	.85	.88	1.36	.94
Lesotho	.85	.84	.86	1.08
Tanzania	.80	.79	1.06	1.35
Lusaka	.77	.94	1.10	na
Mauritius	1.07	1.09	1.31	1.07
Manila	1.01	1.23	2.56	na
Singapore	2.00	1.87	1.78	na
Sri Lanka	1.22	1.39	na	1.29
Thailand	1.00	1.00	.95	.95
Rio de Janeiro	.90	.91	1.41	na

months. The figure is restricted to the seven surveys where sufficient numbers of men (20 or more) reported multiple sex partners. A clearer link between behaviour and perceived risk is evident in the case of number of partners than was observed for use of condoms. In all seven surveys, there is an unmistakable decline in the proportion feeling themselves to be at no risk, as the number of partners rises. This decline is most pronounced in Thailand and least apparent in Lusaka. The link between number of partners and perceived risk was assessed statistically for all 16 surveys. The null hypothesis was that the proportions reporting that they were at no risk of HIV/AIDS did not vary by number of reported partners. The alternative hypothesis was that this proportion decreased with increasing number of reported partners. In twelve of the surveys, the null hypothesis was rejected (p < 0.05), using a chi-square test for trend. Nevertheless, it should be stressed that, even among men with five or more non-regular or commercial partners in the last 12 months, substantial proportions, ranging from 15 per cent in Côte d'Ivoire to about 50 per cent in Lusaka and Singapore, nevertheless perceive no personal risk of HIV infection.

A preliminary analysis is given in Table 6.3 of socio-demographic differentials in the proportion of all respondents (confined to those aware of AIDS) who feel a moderate or high personal susceptibility to infection. Four key variables have been selected: current age, current marital status, level of schooling, and urban-rural residence. Each of these explanatory, or background factors, has been dichotomized and proportionate differences (akin to relative risks) between the two categories are shown in the table. For instance, the result for Sri Lanka in the left hand column is 1.22, indicating that respondents under the age of 25 are 22 per cent more likely to feel a moderate or high personal risk than respondents aged between 25 and 49 years. In the same column, the result for Tanzania is .80, indicating that, in this country, younger respondents are 20 per cent less likely than older respondents to feel moderate or high risk. It should be noted that the results pertain to respondents of both sexes, as analyses show few substantial differences in personal risk perceptions between men and women.

The general impression from Table 6.3 is that socio-demographic differentials tend to be modest: proportionate differences are typically no more than 20 per cent (i.e. 1.20 to .80). With regard to age differences, there appears to be a general tendency for older respondents to feel more at risk, though all differences are modest. In Singapore and Sri Lanka, the opposite is found but, in both cases, absolute differences are not great: Singapore, 6.4 versus 3.2 per cent; Sri Lanka 7.1 versus 5.8 per cent. Singapore and Sri Lanka are again the only marked exceptions to the generalization that risk perceptions are broadly similar among the never-married as among those currently in a stable partnership.

Sero-surveillance results suggest HIV prevalence is usually much higher in urban than in rural areas. Accordingly, it might be anticipated that there would be a parallel difference in feelings of personal risk. These expectations receive little empirical support. In only two out of the eleven surveys, in which both urban and rural strata are represented, is there an appreciable divergence in risk perception. In Côte d'Ivoire, 52 per cent of urban respondents, but only 37 per cent of rural respondents, reported moderate or high risk; in Tanzania the corresponding figures are 22 and 16 per cent. In Sri Lanka, the relative difference is also large but the absolute difference is trivial (7.1 versus 5.5 per cent).

The educational background of respondents emerges as a stronger predictor of risk perception than place of residence. In all but three surveys, men or women with secondary or higher schooling are more likely to feel a personal vulnerability to AIDS than those with primary or no schooling. The educational contrast is particularly marked in Singapore, Manila, Côte d'Ivoire, Guinea Bissau, Kenya and Rio de Janeiro.

In order to investigate more rigorously the predictors of perceived personal risk, multiple regression analyses were performed on a sub-set of six surveys. The regressand variable was converted into a numerical scale with the following values: 1 (no risk), 2 (small risk), 3 (don't know), 4 (moderate) and 5 (high). A total of nine regressor variables was selected on the basis of exploratory analysis. These include the four socio-demographic factors shown in Table 6.3, together with three cognitive, one attitudinal and one behavioural variable. The cognitive variables are: belief in casual transmission, belief in sexual transmission, and belief in transmission by an asymptomatic HIV-sufferer. There are good common sense grounds for expecting that the sense of personal risk might be related to each of these beliefs. In particular, belief in casual transmission, shown to be widespread in Chapter 3, might well engender a heightened sense of vulnerability. These variables are represented as yes/no dichotomies in the regression models. Risk behaviour is also represented as a dichotomy; individuals who reported any sexual contacts outside of regular partnerships in the preceding 12 months are distinguished from all other respondents. The last variable to be included is perceived threat of AIDS to the health of the community; this is represented as a numerical scale with values ranging from 1 (no threat at all) to 4 (serious threat).

Multiple regression on perceived personal risk was run for males and females separately. All first-order interactive effects between the nine predictor variables were systematically screened for statistical significance. Tables 6.4(a) and (b) provide an initial overview of results, by showing which predictor variables have statistically significant ($p < 0.05$) main or interactive net effects on perceived personal risk.

Perhaps the most striking result is the general absence of a link between beliefs about HIV transmission and perceived personal risk. In no survey that gathered the relevant information does a belief in sexual transmission or asymptomatic transmission emerge as a significant predictor, net of other variables in the model. Belief in casual transmission is found to be a significant predictor in three out of the ten regressions: for males in Lusaka and Thailand and for females in Côte d'Ivoire. In each case, the effect is in the expected direction: individuals who believe in casual transmission feel greater personal vulnerability. These mixed results preclude any simple generalizations about the relevance of erroneous beliefs concerning transmission to perceived vulnerability. In most populations they have no impact. In a minority of settings, however, they do lead to an increased sense of personal risk.

Reported sexual behaviour is significantly associated with perceived personal risk in four male and three female study populations. The results are shown in Table 6.5, in terms of adjusted scores. In each of these populations, those who report any non-regular or commercial sex in the preceding twelve months have a higher score, indicating greater perceived vulnerability to HIV/AIDS. Differences, though statistically significant, are not as large in the three African populations as in Thailand. In Rio de Janeiro, there was a significant interaction between risk behaviour and education among male respondents. The effect of risk behaviour on perceived risk was found to be greater among the uneducated than among the educated. This somewhat unexpected finding may reflect greater condom use among educated men.

The technique of multiple regression allows us to reassess relationships between socio-demographic characteristics and perceived risk, net of the possibly confounding effects of other variables. In the earlier bivariate analysis (Table 6.3), respondents' age was only weakly related to risk in most surveys. The results of the multiple regression, however, indicate significant effects in nine of the 12 populations. One reason for this apparent discrepancy is that age was dichotomized in the earlier analysis but is introduced into regressions in the form of five groups. The pattern of the relationships

Table 6.4(a): Summary of results of multiple regression analyses on perceived personal risk among men

Predictors	Côte d'Ivoire	Burundi	Lusaka	Manila	Thailand	Rio de Janeiro
Age	*	*	*	*	–	–
Education	*	*	–	–	*	*
Marital status	*	–	–	–	*	–
Residence	–	–	na	na	–	na
Belief in casual transmission	–	–	*	–	*	–
Belief in sexual transmission	na	–	–	–	–	–
Belief in asymptomatic transmission	na	–	–	–	–	na
Reported risk behaviour	*	–	*	–	*	x
Perceived threat	na	*	–	*	–	na
Interaction: risk behaviour education	–	–	–	–	–	*

Notes: * Enters model as main variable (p < 0.05)
 x Enters model as interaction
 na Data not available

Table 6.4(b): Summary of results of multiple regression analyses on perceived personal risk among women

Predictors	Côte d'Ivoire	Burundi	Lusaka	Manila	Thailand	Rio de Janeiro
Age	*	–	*	*	*	*
Education	*	*	–	–	–	–
Marital status	–	*	*	*	*	–
Residence	*	–	na	na	–	na
Belief in casual transmission	*	–	–	–	–	–
Belief in sexual transmission	na	–	–	–	–	–
Belief in asymptomatic transmission	na	–	–	–	–	na
Reported risk behaviour	*	–	–	–	*	*
Perceived threat	na	*	–	*	–	na

Notes: * Enters model as main effect (p < 0.05)
 na Data not available

Table 6.5: Net effects of reported sexual behaviour on perceived personal risk

Study Group		Adjusted Scores		
		No-risk behaviour	Risk behaviour	Difference
Côte d'Ivoire	Males	2.77	3.08	0.31
Côte d'Ivoire	Females	2.53	2.76	0.23
Lusaka	Males	2.24	2.63	0.39
Thailand	Males	1.70	2.43	0.73
Thailand	Females	1.84	2.40	0.56
Rio de Janeiro	Males – No education	2.00	3.12	1.12
Rio de Janeiro	Males – Some education	2.35	2.71	0.36
Rio de Janeiro	Females	2.33	2.72	0.39

is similar in all but one population. Perceived risk is highest in the inter-mediate age groups, in part perhaps a reflection that some of the younger respondents are still sexually inexperienced. As shown in Chapter 4, risk behaviour tends to peak in the middle age groups. Women in Rio de Janeiro are the exception; among this population, perceived risk rises monotonically with age, a reflection of late marriage and little premarital sex for women.

Current marital status is more likely to be a predictor of perceived risk among women than men. In Burundi and Lusaka, women who are in a current partnership, or were formerly married, express more vulnerability to AIDS than never-married women. In Côte d'Ivoire, the other African country selected for multivariate analysis, the difference is in the same direction but it is not statistically significant. The same pattern holds for Thailand, suggest-ing that fear of infection by the husband may be common. In Manila, how-ever, the opposite result is obtained; in this city, single women express the greatest personal risk. This result is not readily explicable because few single women in Manila report risk behaviour, nor is belief in casual transmission a significant predictor.

The effects of place of residence can only be examined for three of the six surveys selected for multivariate analysis. In only one group, women of the Côte d'Ivoire, is a statistically significant result found, thus confirming the impression of the earlier bivariate analysis. The effects of education, that were pronounced in the bivariate analysis, attenuate when other factors are controlled. Nevertheless, net effects remain significant in four of the six male populations and in two of the female populations. Typically, respondents with secondary or higher schooling express the highest perceived risk. Among Côte d'Ivoire males, however, adjusted results suggest that risk perception is highest among those with no schooling. In Thailand, the relationship be-tween level of schooling and risk perception score is negative and widens, rather than narrows, after controlling for other variables in the model. The situation among the male population of Rio de Janeiro is more complicated because of an interaction between schooling and risk behaviour. As shown in Table 6.5, educated men who report no risk behaviour in the last twelve months are more likely to feel vulnerable to AIDS than corresponding un-educated men. But among those reporting sexual contacts outside of regular partnerships, the differential is reversed. As mentioned earlier, greater use of condoms by educated men in Rio de Janeiro may be part of the explanation.

Behavioural Change

As mentioned at the start of this chapter, behavioural change is one of the most important topics included in KABP and PR surveys. Pending the discov-ery of an effective vaccine or therapy, reduction of risk-carrying behaviours is the only way in which the spread of the pandemic will be arrested. In this

Table 6.6: *Among those aware of AIDS, the percentage who think that a person can avoid HIV/AIDS through behavioural change*

Survey	Males	Females
Central African Republic	89	86
Côte d'Ivoire	86	69
Guinea Bissau	66	56
Togo	85	75
Burundi	93	87
Kenya	72	69
Lesotho	89	91
Tanzania	88	87
Lusaka	89	87
Mauritius	83	74
Manila	61	57
Singapore	69	71
Sri Lanka	46	41
Thailand	94	91

section, responses to four questions on behavioural change are analyzed. This cluster of questions came late in the interview, immediately following items on perceived threat of AIDS and perceived personal risk. By the time they were posed, respondents to KABP surveys had been exposed to some fifteen minutes of questioning on AIDS-related knowledge and sources of information. In PR surveys, respondents, in addition, had answered a battery of questions about their own sexual behaviour. As we shall see, interpretation of responses has to take into account the context in which they were administered.

The purpose of the first question on behavioural change – *Can a person avoid AIDS by changing his/her behaviour? That is by doing certain things and not doing other things?* – was to assess whether or not respondents felt able to influence by their own actions their chances of infection. This dimension of subjective efficacy is a key element in some theories of health behaviour (e.g. Rotter, 1966; Ajzen, 1988). To the extent that persons feel that their future is determined by forces outside their control (e.g. an external locus of control), the chance that they will make appropriate behavioural responses to threats is reduced.

Table 6.6 shows the percentage of respondents who gave a positive response, thereby indicating a sense of subjective efficacy with regard to HIV infection. The outstanding feature is the high percentages in most surveys who think that behavioural change can be effective. In all the African surveys, substantial majorities answered positively; this pattern lends no support to the earlier speculation that superstitious or magical beliefs about transmission might be more common in west and central Africa than elsewhere.

Among the non-African surveys, the results are more mixed. In Mauritius and Thailand, large majorities think that people can avoid AIDS by behavioural change, but the proportions are appreciably lower in Manila, Singapore and Sri Lanka. As these populations are highly educated this pattern is unexpected. In Sri Lanka, however, detailed knowledge about transmission of HIV was rather poor; and in all three settings, the number of reported AIDS cases was very low at the time of the surveys. Perhaps a feeling that behavioural change was not needed has influenced answers to this question.

A second important feature of Table 6.6 is the generally modest difference in response between men and women. To the extent that women feel less able, for a variety of reasons, to control risk of infection via their male partners, we might have expected a large divide in attitude between men and women. While in most surveys, men are more likely to express a sense of subjective efficacy than women, the differences are small (i.e. less than ten per cent), with only three exceptions: Côte d'Ivoire, Guinea Bissau and Togo.

We turn now to consider reporting of behavioural changes in response to the threat of AIDS. Respondents were asked, *Have you made any changes in your behaviour or way of life as a result of what you have learned about AIDS?* The key results, in Figure 6.6, show a surprisingly high reporting of behavioural change. Among the African populations, over half of all men claim to have changed their behaviour to reduce the risk of HIV infection. This proportion exceeds 80 per cent in the Central African Republic and is over seventy per cent in Côte d'Ivoire, Guinea Bissau and Togo. Thus it is in central and west Africa that the most emphatically positive results are found. In east and southern Africa, over 60 per cent of males in Lesotho, Tanzania and Lusaka report change; 50 per cent in Burundi and Kenya report change.

Among the non-African sites, reported behavioural change corresponds more closely to the level of HIV infection. Where the epidemic is at a very early stage (Mauritius, Manila, Singapore and Sri Lanka), small minorities of men report change. In Thailand and Rio de Janeiro, where the epidemic was at a more advanced phase at the time of the surveys, behavioural change is more common among men: 60 per cent in Thailand and 40 per cent in Rio de Janeiro.

Figure 6.6 also shows the proportion of men and women who say that they have not modified their behaviour but respond affirmatively to the question *Do you intend to make any changes in the future?* In all surveys, these proportions are small compared to the figures for actual change. Indeed the proportions who have not made but intend to make changes in their behaviour are below 10 per cent, except in Guinea Bissau and Lesotho (15 and 12 per cent, respectively).

Are women as likely as men to report behavioural change in response to AIDS? In view of the fact that they are much less likely to admit sexual risk behaviour than men, the expected answer is negative and Figure 6.6 confirms that this is indeed the case. Table 6.7 summarizes sex differentials in reported change. With the single exception of Lesotho, more men report change than women. In the Central African Republic, the difference is trivially small and, in Guinea Bissau and Lusaka, it is modest. For Lesotho, the results are consistent with reporting of risk behaviours. In this country, an atypically high proportion of women admitted sex with non-regular partners

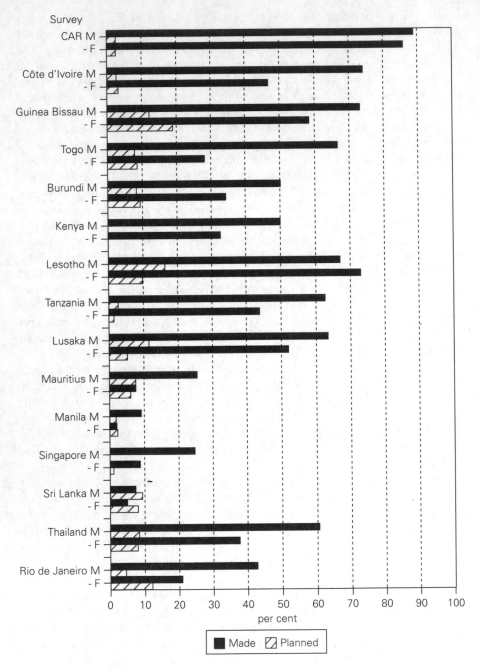

Figure 6.6: Percentage of male (M) and female (F) respondents who report that they have: a) made; b) plan to make behavioural change (restricted to those aware of AIDS)

Table 6.7: Number of men who reported behavioural change per 100 women reporting change

	Number
Central African Republic	103
Côte d'Ivoire	158
Guinea Bissau	125
Togo	238
Burundi	146
Kenya	153
Lesotho	92
Tanzania	143
Zambia	122
Mauritius	327
Manila	427
Singapore	281
Sri Lanka	151
Thailand	160
Rio de Janeiro	206

in the preceding 12 months (see Chapter 4). This is not true, however, for the Central African Republic, Lusaka or Guinea Bissau.

In other surveys, the ratio of male to female reporting of change ranges from about 1.5 (in Côte d'Ivoire, Burundi, Kenya, Tanzania, Sri Lanka, and Thailand) to much higher levels in Togo, Mauritius, Manila, Singapore and Rio de Janeiro. The results for Mauritius, Manila, Singapore and Rio de Janeiro are to be expected in view of the very low reporting of risk behaviours by females.

On the basis of rationalistic theories of human behaviour, behavioural change in response to AIDS should be, in part, the consequence of a sense of personal vulnerability to infection. The relationship between these factors is examined in Figure 6.7, which shows the percentage who report change among three perceived vulnerability categories: low, small and moderate or high risk. For clarity of exposition, respondents who were uncertain about personal vulnerability have been omitted.

Among the non-African study populations, there is a pronounced gradient in the expected direction for men. For instance, only 22 per cent of Singaporean males who consider themselves to be at no risk report that they have modified their behaviour; this proportion rises to 40 among those who perceive a small risk and further to 67 per cent for those reporting a moderate or high risk. Among the *uncertain – don't know* category, 30 per cent report behavioural change, implying that uncertainty is similar to low risk in its behavioural implications. This same correspondence holds in most surveys.

There tends to be a less pronounced effect of perceived personal risk on behavioural change among females in the non-African surveys, though differences are in the expected direction. This is to be anticipated because, for women more than men, the feeling of vulnerability is presumably more likely

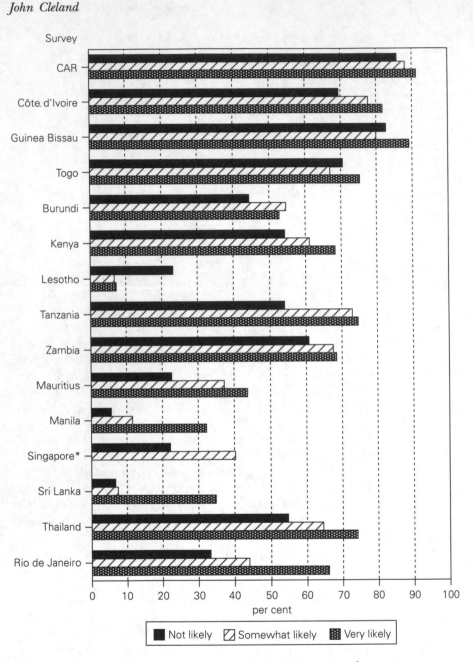

Note: results not shown for *very likely* category because there are too few cases

Figure 6.7(a): Percentage of male respondents who have reported that they have made behavioural change, by perceived personal risk of AIDS (restricted to those aware of AIDS)

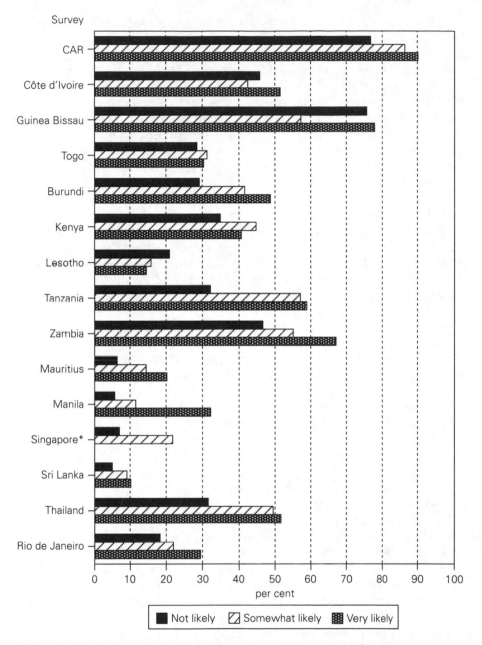

Note: results not shown for very likely category because there are too few cases

Figure 6.7(b): Percentage of female respondents who have reported that they have made behavioural change, by perceived personal risk of AIDS (restricted to those aware of AIDS)

to stem from worries about the behaviour of regular partners than from their own behaviour.

The pattern of results for the African surveys is somewhat different. The relationship between perceived risk and reported behavioural change is rather weak. In other words, those who say that they feel little or no personal risk of HIV infection are almost as likely to report a modification of behaviour as those who feel a high risk. The results for Lusaka illustrate the point; the percentages reporting behavioural shifts rise from 61 to 68 and to 69 per cent across the three categories of perceived risk: an extremely modest increase. One possible reason is that respondents who have changed their behaviour now report little or no risk; in other words, low risk perception at the time of the survey reflects past behaviour change. Logical though this may be, it is not a plausible explanation. Behavioural risk reduction is typically a matter of degree rather than a more radical elimination of risk behaviour; thus those who report a change are unlikely to feel themselves free of risk nor is it plausible that changes in behaviour have occurred on a scale implied by the testimonies of African respondents. Finally, it is difficult to invoke an explanation for the African surveys that does not apply elsewhere.

A more likely explanation of the weak link between perceived risk and reported behavioural change in most of the African surveys is that the latter response should not be interpreted literally but rather taken as a verbal assent to a general need for, or desirability of change (i.e. a normative response given in the context of an interview about a serious and frightening disease).

Problems of interpretation become more severe when behavioural change is classified by sexual behaviour reported in the last 12 months. Figure 6.8 shows the proportion of men who reported change among the same four behavioural risk groupings used in Figure 6.4. The difficulty of interpretation arises from the fact that we do not know the extent to which behaviour in the last 12 months reflects any changes that have been made. Nor do we always know whether any change concerns sexual behaviour.

The most common pattern in Figure 6.8 takes the form of a positive association between reported risk behaviour in the recent past and reported changes in behaviour. Thus men who have been at greater risk of HIV transmission are more likely to claim a change in behaviour. The obvious interpretation is that reported change has only been partial or that it indicates a perceived need or readiness to change rather than achievement of change. This pattern is most clear-cut in the non-African surveys. In Singapore, for instance, 64 per cent of men who reported contact with sex workers in the last 12 months claimed some behavioural change, compared to only about 20 per cent of men who restricted any sexual experience to regular partnerships.

Among the African surveys, the relationship between past behaviour and change is more varied. In some settings (Lesotho, Lusaka, Togo), there is no pronounced link. In Kenya and Tanzania, however, the differences are large with a pattern similar to that found in the non-African surveys.

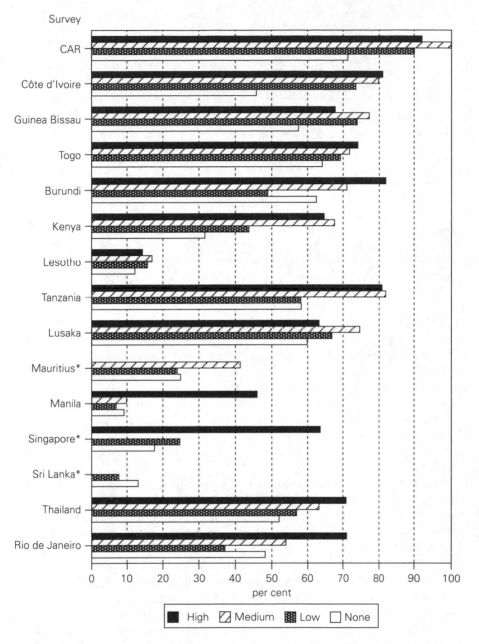

Note: results not shown for all risk categories because there are too few cases

Figure 6.8: *Percentage of male respondents who have reported that they have made behavioural change, by risk behaviour in the last 12 months (restricted to those aware of AIDS)*

Table 6.8: Socio-demographic differentials in proportions of male (M) and female (F) respondents who report behavioural change

Survey	Age less than 25 vs. 25–49 (=1.00)		Never-married vs. Currently Married (=1.00)		Secondary+ School vs. Primary or No School (=1.00)		Urban vs. Rural (=1.00)	
	M	F	M	F	M	F	M	F
CAR	.98	1.04	.87	.98	1.02	1.04	.98	1.05
Côte d'Ivoire	.99	1.23	.86	.89	1.14	1.38	1.00	.93
Guinea Bissau	1.03	1.13	1.04	1.20	1.35	1.64	1.10	1.47
Togo	.91	1.54	.94	1.27	1.22	1.18	1.06	.92
Burundi	1.08	1.09	1.01	.90	1.50	1.52	1.46	1.87
Kenya	1.07	1.51	1.04	1.55	1.25	1.11	.80	.99
Lesotho	1.15	.96	.90	.82	1.13	1.06	.94	1.01
Tanzania	.98	.93	1.02	.89	1.07	1.07	1.19	1.47
Lusaka	1.05	1.03	.91	.78	1.05	.91	–	–
Mauritius	.85	1.25	1.08	1.24	1.02	.97	.86	.93
Manila	1.79	2.00	1.77	3.70	.87	1.00	–	–
Singapore	.76	1.46	.97	1.53	.78	2.66	–	–
Sri Lanka	1.15	.94	.89	.63	–	–	.71	.71
Thailand	1.00	1.09	1.06	1.10	1.00	1.21	.98	.95
Rio de Janeiro	1.06	1.05	1.11	1.29	1.25	1.45	–	–

Table 6.8 provides a preliminary analysis of socio-demographic differentials in the proportion of all respondents (among those aware of AIDS) who report any behavioural change. The Table shows proportionate differences, as in Table 6.3 on perceived risk. Differences in the propensity to report change between younger and older men are generally modest, except in Manila where 13 per cent of those under 25 years say that they have modified behaviour compared to only 7 per cent of older men. For women, age differences are more likely to be pronounced. In Togo, Kenya, Mauritius, Manila, and Singapore, younger respondents are appreciably more likely to report change than older respondents.

With regard to marital status, there is considerable variation both in the direction and magnitude of differences. As with current age, contrasts are more marked for women than for men. In most of the non-African surveys, single women are more likely to report change than married women, but Sri Lanka proves to be an exception. In the African surveys, the prevailing pattern is for change to be more concentrated among the married than the unmarried, but there are several exceptions (e.g. Kenya, Togo). For men, marital status makes little difference to the reporting of change. With only one outlier, all differences fall within the range of .80 to 1.20.

In the earlier analysis of perceived personal risk, urban-rural residence proved to be an erratic and weak predictor. The same is true with regard to behavioural change. Among the 22 sex-specific study populations for which an urban–rural breakdown is possible, higher levels of change are reported in urban areas in ten instances but lower levels in twelve. Moreover, differences are small except in Burundi and Sri Lanka.

Respondents' education exerts a positive influence on behavioural change. There are only two exceptions for men and three minor ones for women. In all other study populations, individuals with secondary schooling are more likely to report change than individuals with primary or no schooling.

Thus far in the discussion, the nature of the changes that respondents claim to have made has been ignored. This omission is remedied in Table 6.9. The model KABP and PR questionnaires allowed for the recording of verbatim answers to the question, *What changes have you made?* It was recommended that a maximum of three answers be coded. In several surveys, however, only one answer was coded. In many other surveys, the number of second or third answers is small. Hence the analysis in Table 6.9 is restricted to the first (and usually the most important) change mentioned by respondents.

It is not always possible to infer the meaning behind coded responses in some surveys. Typical of such problematic codes are *avoid strangers* and *be more careful.* These have been classified in table 6.9 as ambiguous (column 7). They account for substantial minorities of replies in the Central African Republic, Côte d'Ivoire, Kenya and Mauritius.

In the majority of surveys, the dominant reported change took the form of a reduction in sexual contacts or greater care in choosing partners. Typical answers were *avoid sex with strangers, reduce number of partners, greater faithfulness, avoid prostitutes, sexual abstinence* and *greater care in choosing partners.* Leaving aside the ambiguous reasons, various attempts to reduce the risk of sexual transmission is the most common type of answer in all surveys – apart from Sri Lanka and among women in Mauritius, Manila and Thailand. By comparison, greater use of condoms (column 2) is mentioned by disappointingly few respondents; typically less than 10 per cent report this type of change and the number is close to zero in several surveys. Moreover, as discussed in Chapter 2, there are grounds for doubting the validity of responses; appreciable proportions of those claiming greater use of condoms had reported earlier that they had never used this device. The exceptions here are Guinea Bissau, Sri Lanka and Rio de Janeiro.

The salience of sexual behaviour as the main behavioural response to AIDS is further confirmed by considering the number of answers that make mention of drugs or needles, or of receiving or donating blood (columns 3 and 4). In most surveys, very few respondents reported such changes in behaviour. The main exceptions are Burundi (where a somewhat astonishing 28 per cent of women said they had avoided *syringes*), Tanzania, and females in Thailand and Rio de Janeiro.

Of special interest is the number of people who report changes that imply a belief in casual transmission (e.g. eating alone, avoiding public toilets, not sharing clothes, not touching strangers, avoiding travel, avoiding barbers). In view of the substantial proportion of respondents who believe in casual transmission of HIV, or are unsure, surprisingly few behavioural changes fall in this category (column 5). The proportion is close to zero in most groups and less than 10 per cent in all groups, except males and females in Manila. Similarly, proportions saying that they have improved general health

Table 6.9: Among respondents who have made changes, percentage mentioning specific changes

Survey	1 Sex	2 Condoms	3 Drugs	4 Blood	5 Casual	6 Health	7 Other ambiguous	8 DK	N
CAR									
Males	55	4	0	0	0	0	38	3	962
Females	75	1	0	0	0	0	22	4	780
All	63	3	0	0	0	0	31	3	1742
Côte d'Ivoire									
Males	59	6	0	0	0	1	22	12	1049
Females	57	3	0	0	0	5	21	14	606
All	58	5	6	0	0	3	22	12	1655
Guinea Bissau									
Males	45	25	4	1	2	3	4	16	481
Females	63	17	4	0	4	2	6	4	190
All	50	23	4	1	2	3	3	14	671
Togo									
Males	82	0	2	0	6	2	5	3	559
Females	66	1	0	1	8	8	11	5	187
All	78	0	1	0	7	3	6	5	746
Burundi									
Males	70	0	8	0	0	0	0	22	555
Females	52	0	28	0	0	0	0	20	367
All	63	0	16	0	0	0	0	21	922
Kenya									
Males	49	1	1	1	1	0	34	13	584
Females	37	1	3	2	1	0	45	11	490
All	44	1	2	2	1	0	39	11	1074
Tanzania									
Males	81	7	12	0	0	0	0	0	1118
Females	83	4	14	0	0	0	0	1	970
All	82	5	13	0	0	0	0	1	2088
Mauritius									
Males	21	1	0	0	7	5	40	25	302
Females	10	0	2	0	11	12	23	42	84
All	18	1	1	0	8	7	36	29	386
Manila									
Males	39	0	0	0	15	0	7	39	59
Females	10	0	0	0	19	10	5	56	21
All	31	0	0	0	16	3	6	44	80
Singapore									
Males	68	4	0	0	3	4	0	21	243
Females	31	4	1	0	8	7	0	49	91
All	58	4	0	0	5	5	0	28	334
Sri Lanka									
Males	7	20	0	0	0	0	0	73	89
Females	11	18	0	0	0	0	0	71	55
All	8	19	0	0	0	0	0	73	144
Thailand									
Males	53	6	2	1	0	0	0	38	678
Females	14	3	13	1	0	0	0	69	629
All	34	4	7	1	0	0	0	54	1307
Rio de Janeiro									
Males	65	18	2	1	4	2	1	7	253
Females	34	10	16	1	5	9	10	15	147
All	54	15	7	1	3	4	4	12	406

Note: see text for discussion of the type of changes

precautions (e.g. better food, more exercise, greater hygiene) as a means of avoiding AIDS are very small (see column 6). The general conclusion is clear-cut. Among respondents who report behavioural modification, most mention changes that appear to be potentially effective forms of risk reduction.

As a final step in the analysis of behavioural change, logistic regression analysis was performed. The dependent variable was reporting of *effective* behavioural change. To construct this variable, respondents were dichotomized. The first category comprises those who reported a change that was considered to be potentially effective at reducing the risk of HIV infection. The four main types of effective change correspond to column 1 to 4 of Table 6.9, namely reduced sexual activity or great circumspection, increased condom use, avoidance of drugs and injections, and of unhygienic blood transfers. All other respondents – those who reported no change or a change classified as ineffective or ambiguous – form the second category. A total of nine predictor variables was selected. These are almost identical to those used in the previous multivariate analysis of perceived personal risk. The latter variable now appears as a predictor rather than as a outcome variable. Regressions were restricted to respondents who were aware of AIDS and had some experience of sexual intercourse. Although it can be argued that those who are not yet sexually active should be included because the maintenance of virginity may itself be a response to the threat of HIV, it was felt that the results of the regression would have greater interpretability if such respondents were excluded.

These results are summarized in Tables 6.10a and b. Considering the findings for males first, it is worth noting several negative features. Beliefs in different modes of transmission are unrelated to the likelihood of behavioural change in any of the sub-set of six surveys. Current age is a significant predictor only in Lusaka. More surprisingly, education is also a predictor of change in one country only: Côte d'Ivoire. The presence of perceived personal risk in the model may account for this negative finding. As noted earlier, educated respondents tend to perceive greater risk of infection than uneducated respondents and risk itself is a strong predictor of change. Among four of the six study groups, perceived personal risk has a significant effect on reported change, net of all other factors. The results in terms of adjusted percentages are shown in Table 6.11. As may be seen, the precise nature of the relationships take a variety of forms. In Côte d'Ivoire and Rio de Janeiro, there is a monotonic increase in the likelihood of reported change with each increment in perceived risk, leading to substantial differences across the spectrum. In Manila, however, the only significant difference lies between those who report no risk and all others.

Sexual risk behaviour is related to change in only two of the male study groups, Manila and Rio de Janeiro. In both instances, men who report sex outside of regular partnerships in the preceding 12 months are also more likely to claim to have modified their behaviour than those who report no such casual or commercial sex.

Table 6.10(a): Summary of results of log linear regressions on reporting of (effective) behavioural change among men

Predictors	Côte d'Ivoire	Burundi	Lusaka	Manila	Thailand	Rio
Age	–	–	*	–	–	–
Education	*	–	–	–	–	–
Marital Status	*	–	*	–	*	*
Residence	–	*	na	na	*	na
Belief in casual transmission	–	–	–	–	–	–
Belief in asymptomatic transmission	na	–	–	–	na	na
Reported risk behaviour	–	–	–	*	–	*
Personal risk	*	–	–	*	*	*
Perceived threat	na	–	–	–	na	na

Notes: * Enters model as main variable ($p < 0.05$)
na Data not available

Table 6.10(b): Summary of results of log linear regressions on reporting of effective behavioural change among women

Predictors	Côte d'Ivoire	Burundi	Lusaka	Manila	Thailand	Rio
Age	*	–	–	–	–	*
Education	*	*	*	–	–	–
Marital Status	–	–	*	*	–	–
Residence	–	–	na	na	–	na
Belief in casual transmission	–	*	–	–	–	–
Belief in asymptomatic transmission	na	*	–	–	na	na
Reported risk behaviour	*	–	–	–	*	*
Personal risk	*	*	–	*	–	–
Perceived threat	na	*	–	–	na	na

Notes: * Enters model as main variable ($p < 0.05$)
na Data not available

Table 6.11: Adjusted percentage of respondents reporting effective change, by degree of risk perception

	Perceived risk				
	Low (1)	2	3	4	High 5
Males					
Côte d'Ivoire	42	46	50	55	59
Manila	5	17	17	17	17
Thailand	35	35	44	44	44
Rio de Janeiro	34	38	42	47	52
Females					
Côte d'Ivoire	28	28	28	28	40
Burundi	10	–	12	15	18
Manila	2	2	4	6	8

Among men, behavioural change varies significantly according to current marital status in four of the six groups. In Côte d'Ivoire, married men are more likely to report change than the never married or formerly married. In Lusaka, Thailand and Rio de Janeiro, this differential is reversed. Finally we may note that place of residence predicts change in Burundi and Thailand. In the former country, urban men are more likely to report change, but adjusted differences are not large (10 versus 6 per cent). In Thailand, it is rural respondents who claim a higher level of change but again the difference is not marked (39 versus 32 per cent).

The results for women largely parallel those for men. Perceived personal risk is a significant predictor in three cases (see Table 6.10b), as is sexual risk behaviour in the last twelve months. In Thailand and Rio de Janeiro, the adjusted differences by risk behaviour are very large:

		per cent change
Thailand:	risk behaviour	26
	no risk behaviour	7
Rio de Janeiro:	risk behaviour	33
	no risk behaviour	13

For women, education emerges as a stronger net influence on behavioural change than was observed for men. In all three African surveys, educated women are significantly more likely to report a modification in behaviour than uneducated women.

Conclusion and Implications

Whilst governments and communities have often been slow to recognise the seriousness of the AIDS pandemic, this is perhaps not always the case for individuals. A majority of respondents in most surveys spontaneously mentioned this disease as one of the most serious global and national health problems. Even in settings where very few AIDS cases have been reported, such as Mauritius, Singapore, and Manila, there was no widespread denial of the general threat. Moreover, the threat is seen as an increasing one in these sites. However, this finding does not hold for all of African surveys. In the Central African Republic, Togo, Tanzania and Lusaka, there is little appreciation that HIV-related health problems and associated mortality are likely to worsen in the future before they improve. The policy implications of this dissonance between epidemiological probability and public consciousness are not obvious; there is a danger, for instance, that people living in severely affected areas might be numbed into inactivity by the prospect of a worsening situation. Hope is a better spur to action than despair.

The widespread recognition of the general threat of AIDS is paralleled by surprisingly high levels of reported personal vulnerability or risk, both among men and women. In all but one of the African surveys, over half of respondents perceive themselves to be at some risk, or are unsure. The corresponding proportions are much lower in the non-African surveys, except for Rio de Janeiro. The results are surprising when set against information presented in earlier chapters. In Chapter 3, we saw that, in most sites, 90 per cent of respondents (among those aware of AIDS) were knowledgeable about sexual transmission, while the analysis in Chapter 4 showed that the proportions reporting risky sexual behaviour in the preceding 12 months were generally small.

Why then should the sense of personal vulnerability be so prevalent? One obvious explanation is that beliefs in sexual transmission co-exist with beliefs in transmission of HIV by casual contact, as was shown in Chapter 3. However, this hypothesis was not confirmed by the statistical analysis. Belief in casual transmission was not a significant predictor of perceived personal risk in most of the study populations.

Another equally obvious possible explanation is that respondents are aware of the risk of infection via the behaviour of the regular partner rather than via their own behaviour. This factor presumably colours the risk perceptions of women. Women themselves are much less likely than men to report sexual contact outside stable partnerships than men (though there are a few exceptions). Yet, their feelings of vulnerability to HIV infection are similar to those of men. It is probably no coincidence that substantial proportions of women, particularly among the African study populations, are aware that their husbands have other sexual partners (see Chapter 4). Similar feelings among men are far less common (except in Lesotho).

A third possible explanation is that, despite almost universal knowledge of sexual transmission and the fact that belief in casual transmission does not appear to be a relevant factor in most settings, there exists a widely diffuse sense of personal risk that has no obvious rational basis. This characterization is more plausible for the four francophone countries of central and west Africa than elsewhere. The proportions reporting a moderate or high personal risk are much higher in this sub-region than elsewhere. Furthermore, the links between perception of vulnerability and reported risk behaviours are weak; even persons who report no sexual activity at all in the preceding twelve months are almost as likely to express feelings of personal risk as those who report commercial or casual sex.

One of the long term goals of public information campaigns is to instill among citizens realistic perceptions of risk. Individuals who have unprotected intercourse outside of mutually faithful partnerships should be aware that their behaviour carries some risk, even though it may be impossible to quantify. Conversely, individuals who are not sexually active or restrict sex to regular partnerships should realize that their behaviour minimizes the chances of HIV infection. On the evidence of these surveys, this goal is far from achieved, particularly in west and central Africa. Even in other settings, the link between reported behaviour and risk perception is not strong. In most of the study populations, perceived risk rises significantly in step with number of sexual partners in the last 12 months. But even among men who report five or more partners (outside of marriage), a substantial number, ranging from 20 to 50 per cent, perceive no risk to themselves. Protection by condoms is no explanation for this result, because it is still rarely practised in most of the study sites. Nor does regular condom use necessarily engender a greater sense of safety against infection. One of the many surprising results contained in this chapter is that, in only two of seven surveys for which statistical analysis was feasible, did regular use of condoms in commercial sex encounters apparently lead to a reduced sense of risk among men. The policy indication is obvious and reinforces the message contained elsewhere in this volume: there remains a huge task of popularizing condom use as one method of protection against HIV.

The examination of socio-demographic predictors of perceived vulnerability proved interesting in several regards. Personal perceptions were generally highest in the middle of the age range, a result in concordance with patterns of sexual behaviour. Among women, perceived vulnerability was significantly greater among married than single women in three of the six sites selected for multivariate analysis. This result reinforces the suggestion made earlier that women are likely to fear infection via their regular partners. Educational background emerges as the most consistent positive predictor of perceived personal risk; this pattern runs counter to suspicions that risk perceptions are generally higher than anticipated because the relevant question has been misunderstood. If this were the case, an inverse relationship between educational status and degree of reported risk would have been expected.

The last section of the chapter concerns behavioural change. The most striking feature is the very high proportions of men and women who believe in the efficacy of behavioural change and who claim to have modified their behaviour because of AIDS. Among men aware of AIDS, 50 per cent or more report behavioural modification in all the African surveys. The corresponding proportions for women are appreciably lower but nevertheless exceed 30 per cent in all but one African site. Outside the African subcontinent, changes are reported much less commonly and the pattern corresponds to the stage of the HIV epidemics. Thus in Mauritius, Manila, Singapore and Sri Lanka, with few AIDS cases at the time of the surveys, only minorities report that they have changed their behaviour. In Rio de Janeiro and Thailand, on the other hand, the reported behavioural response is similar to the level in Africa.

A second striking feature of the survey findings is that the dominant expression of change implies a reduction of sexual risk behaviour. Avoid prostitutes, reduce number of partners and showing greater faithfulness are the most common variants of this type of answer. Greater use of condoms is rarely mentioned, except in Guinea Bissau. And few respondents report changes that reflect beliefs in casual transmission or that stem from other erroneous causal attributions.

Were these results to be taken at face value, they would denote a massive swing away from sexual risk behaviours, particularly among African men. However, these responses cannot be viewed as convincing evidence of radical reductions in sexual risk behaviour. There are three main reasons for a much more cautious and sceptical interpretation. First, there is no evidence, for instance, from declines in numbers of sex workers or in the incidence of sexually transmitted diseases, to corroborate the survey findings. Admittedly, adequate studies of these trends are lacking, but it is unlikely that major changes would have gone unnoticed. Second, men who claim to have changed their behaviour are more likely, not less likely, to report commercial or non-regular sex in the last 12 months than men who report no change. While it is logically possible that changes have been too recent to depress aggregate behaviour over the 12-month period, it is more plausible to reach a verdict that changes have been very slight, and even more plausible to reach a tentative conclusion that reported change may signify an acknowledgement of the desirability or need to change rather than its achievement. The third reason for caution concerns the context in which questions on behavioural change were administered, They came towards the end of some 30 minutes of questions about a new and potentially frightening disease. The temptation to respond positively to items on change may have been powerful because, to do otherwise, may have conveyed an impression to the interviewer of irresponsibility or insensitivity.

Despite these cautions, the results are encouraging. Widespread denial of risk or the need to modify behaviour would have yielded a much gloomier prognosis. The WHO/GPA surveys portray a state of public opinion that appears to be conducive to changes in behaviour that would effectively reduce transmission of the disease. This interpretation of the survey data has profound implications for public information campaigns. It implies that an emphasis on preventive change can be maintained without much risk of a counter-reaction or rejection. The findings also suggest that public advocacy of condoms should not be allowed to overshadow messages about faithfulness. Indeed the results presented in this chapter suggest that reduction in number of sexual partners may be a more common response to the threat of AIDS than condom use.

Chapter 7

Risk Factors Related to HIV Transmission: Sexually Transmitted Diseases, Alcohol Consumption and Medically-related Injections

Benoît Ferry

Introduction

In order to widen the range of topics covered in KABP and PR surveys, but bearing in mind local sensitivities and priorities, additional and optional sections of the WHO/GPA questionnaire were suggested. Their inclusion depended on the discretion of the principal investigator at each survey site. In this chapter, an analysis of three such optional sections is presented: sexually transmitted diseases, other than HIV; alcohol consumption; and injecting practices.

Most of the HIV transmission in the developing world takes place through unprotected sexual contact. It is now established that infection of one or both partners with other sexually transmitted diseases (STDs) may be a powerful co-factor in HIV transmission. It is important to study STDs among general populations because the predominant mode of transmission of both HIV infection and other STDs is sexual. Many of the measures for preventing sexual transmission of HIV and STD are the same, as are the target audiences for these interventions. STD clinical services are an important access point for persons at high risk of both HIV and other STDs, not only for diagnosis and treatment but also for education. There is also a strong association between the occurrence of HIV infection and the presence of other STDs, making early diagnosis and effective treatment of STDs an important strategy for the prevention of HIV transmission. Trends in the incidence and prevalence of selected STDs can also be useful early indicators of change in sexual behaviour, and may be easier to monitor than trends in HIV seroprevalence.

STDs make it easier for HIV to pass from one person to another (Wasserheit, 1992). It has been demonstrated that chancroid, syphilis, chlamydia, gonorrhoea, and trichomoniasis may increase the risk of HIV infection by two to nine times. It is therefore important for HIV control that individuals protect themselves against STDs, recognize the symptoms of STD infection promptly and seek effective treatment for them quickly. Very little is known about the incidence of STDs among general populations, partly because an appreciable number of infected persons are unaware of their condition. This is particularly true for women, among whom infections are more likely to be asymptomatic than among men. Thus many people do not seek medical treatment nor are they aware of means of prevention. The main purpose of the optional set of questions on STDs was to measure disease incidence and treatment.

Alcohol consumption is common in many parts of the world. Its ability to diminish inhibitions and self control is well documented. It thus appeared relevant to explore the levels of consumption and to examine links with sexual activity particularly in the form of non-regular and commercial sexual contacts. The underlying expectation is that drinkers are more exposed to sexual risk-related activities.

A relation between alcohol use and sexual risk practices has been reported in various studies (e.g. Paul, *et al.*, 1991). A study in Zimbabwe on the relations between alcohol use and sexual behaviour (Wilson, *et al.*, 1992) showed a strong association between days when alcohol was consumed and sexual intercourse; alcohol consumption was negatively related to condom use during sexual intercourse with non-regular partners; and the vast majority of contacts with sex workers occurred when the man had been drinking. Most of the workers seek their clients in bars.

A very large proportion of the population in the world receives medically related injections every year. Though the risk of HIV transmission through this route is limited, there may be dangers of infection, especially in those countries where sterilized material is not systematically available or used. The purpose of this optional section was to assess the incidence of injecting practices in the populations surveyed, and thus gauge their potential role in HIV transmission.

Sexually Transmitted Diseases

As mentioned earlier, the presence of STDs may increase the likelihood of HIV transmission. The prompt recognition and treatment of STDs may therefore reduce HIV transmission. Many people do not know that they have an STD, but are merely aware of various pains or symptoms. Patients with STDs generally present in acute stages with one of the following symptoms: urethral or vaginal discharge, genital ulcers, lower abdominal pain, and inguinal bubo, or swollen scrotum. The first two are more specific to STDs than abdominal pain or swollen scrotum. In developing countries, most cases of genital ulcers are the result of chancroid or syphilis. These infections are generally less common than STDs that do not cause genital ulcers, such as chlamydia, gonorrhoea and trichomoniasis. New therapeutic approaches, instead of concentrating on the causative agents involved, focus on groups of signs or symptoms. They are particularly useful for two syndromes: urethral discharge in men and genital ulcer diseases in men and women. The syndrome-based approach facilitates the treatment of large numbers of people with limited resources. For a full picture of STDs/HIV related issues and interventions, see Lande (1993).

The true extent of STDs in general populations remains almost unknown and unstudied, because most studies have been based on subpopulations, such as women attending antenatal, family planning or gynaecological clinics, or male patients in STD clinics. Because they are clinic-based, they are not representative of the general population. For this reason, it is particularly interesting to examine data from representative samples of general populations. The GPA/WHO surveys included questions on the following topics: occurrence of STD symptoms in the previous 12 months; lifetime experience of STDs; frequency of medical treatment of STDs; and knowledge of preventive practices. The results comprise a unique set of comparable data from the following surveys that included the relevant optional section: Côte d'Ivoire, Lesotho, Tanzania (PR), Lusaka, Manila, Singapore, Thailand and Rio de Janeiro.

The analysis here is restricted to responses given by men because of the much greater problem of asymptomatic infection among women. To measure the incidence of STDs, two methods were used in the surveys considered here. An indirect approach via symptoms (genital discharge and sores) was used in Côte d'Ivoire, Lesotho and Tanzania, while a more direct approach that enquired about experience of STDs was used in Lusaka, Thailand and Rio de Janeiro.

Genital Discharge and/or Sores in the Last Year

To measure STD occurrence among men using the indirect approach, the following two questions were asked: *In the last year have you noticed any discharge from your penis that lasted a few days? In the last year have you had any sores on your genital or anal area? Discharge* from the penis refers to any unusual genital discharge, whether or not respondents believed that they knew the cause and whether or not the discharge was painful. Sores on the genital/anal area may take a variety of forms, ranging from painful, inflamed areas to minor abrasions which may cause only mild irritation. All types of sores are counted. The possible causes of sores were not ascertained.

The proportion of sexually active men reporting discharge or sores in the last 12 months was about 11 per cent in Côte d'Ivoire, 21 per cent in Lesotho and 8 per cent in Tanzania. The highest proportion was found among men aged 20 to 24: 16, 26 and 10 per cent in each of the above countries, respectively. Marital status had almost no association with the probability of reporting symptoms, but there was a large difference between

Table 7.1: Percentage of sexually active men who reported they had discharge or sores in the last 12 months, by background characteristics

Background Characteristics	Côte d'Ivoire	Lesotho	Tanzania
All	10.8	20.6	7.6
Age			
15–19	13.2	10.3	7.9
20–24	16.0	26.1	10.3
25–39	11.9	21.8	7.4
40–49	5.7	22.9	5.9
50+	2.7	11.1	–
Marital Status			
Currently married	10.5	20.6	7.4
Formerly married	11.6	25.0	4.7
Never married	12.1	20.0	8.7
Risk behaviour			
No or limited risk	6.5	13.7	4.0
Some risk	18.0	25.7	13.3
Number	1403	428	1627

men who reported any sexual contact outside marriage (or regular partnership) and those who did not. For instance, in Côte d'Ivoire 18 per cent of those who reported non-marital sex in the last 12 months had discharge or sores, compared to 7 per cent for those not at risk in this way. In Lesotho comparable figures were 26 versus 14 per cent, and in Tanzania, 13 versus 4 per cent. This consistency enhances confidence both in reporting of sexual behaviour and of STD symptoms.

In a representative survey of the general population aged 15–54 years conducted in the Mwanza region of Tanzania (Mosha, *et al.*, 1993), 14.4 per cent of the male population reported ever having a genital ulcer (GUS), with an annual incidence of 3.6 per cent; and 28 per cent reported ever having a discharge (GDS), with an annual incidence of 6.8 per cent. Summing the two (GUS and/or GDS) during the last year, the annual incidence becomes 9.7 per cent among the male population. The WHO/GPA survey in Tanzania did not collect directly comparable information on annual incidence. Nevertheless the results of the Mwanza and the national WHO/GPA survey are broadly similar.

Lifetime Experience of STDs

Surveys in Lusaka, Thailand and Rio de Janeiro, asked a question on experience of STDs at any time in the respondent's life. Obviously, the answers are vulnerable to recall lapse particularly for older men. The relevant question was straightforward: *Have you ever had an STD?*

In Lusaka 23 per cent, in Thailand 38 per cent, in Rio de Janeiro 29 per cent of sexually active men reported at least one occurrence of an STD

Table 7.2: Percentage of sexually active men who reported they ever had an STD, by background characteristics

Background Characteristics	Lusaka	Thailand	Rio de Janeiro
All	22.8	37.5	28.7
Age			
15–19	5.4	28.8	4.1
20–24	21.4	39.7	20.5
25–39	30.5	39.5	30.6
40–49	22.1	33.8	38.8
50+	6.6	–	–
Marital Status			
Currently married	25.0	35.1	30.5
Formerly married	21.8	50.0	47.4
Never married	14.0	45.6	20.6
Risk behaviour			
No or limited risk	18.4	28.2	24.8
Some risk	40.2	55.6	38.8
Number	902	895	567

during the course of their lives. For men between the ages of 25–29, these proportions reached 31 per cent in Lusaka, 40 per cent in Thailand, and 31 per cent in Rio de Janeiro. Thus, in these sites, about a third of sexually active adult men reported that they have ever had an STD in their lives.

The link between STDs and sexual risk behaviour is again strong. For example, 40 per cent reporting non-marital sex in the last 12 months in Lusaka also reported having had one or more STDs. The equivalent figures are 56 per cent in Thailand and 39 per cent in Rio de Janeiro. Thus, up to or exceeding one-half of men with a recent history of sexual contact outside marriage have been infected with an STD at least once in their lifetime. These results are particularly difficult to compare with external sources of information about STD incidence or life-time prevalence, because of their unusual nature. Most studies on STDs do not provide any information on levels of infection among the general population. However, in the Mwanza study mentioned earlier, clinical tests were done to measure syphilis (Barongo, et al., 1992). They showed that about 15 per cent of men aged 15–54 years had ever had syphilis and about 8 per cent were currently infected. Another study done in Yaoundé (Cameroon) and Libreville (Gabon) (Sokal, et al., 1992) indicates that the percentages of male secondary students who report ever having had an STD are 10 per cent for ages 15–17, 23 per cent for ages 18–19 and 30 per cent for ages 20–22.

Response to Infection

Two dimensions of response to infection were investigated. In the three surveys that enquired about STD symptoms in the last 12 months, men responding positively were asked: *Were you given medical treatment for any of these conditions in the last 12 months?* The second dimension concerns whether the man informed his partner about the infection and/or took any steps to prevent transmission to her. This line of enquiry was adopted in the three surveys that used the direct, lifetime approach to STD measurement.

In Côte d'Ivoire and Tanzania more than 80 per cent of the men who experienced discharges or sores in the last 12 months were given medical treatment. This proportion falls to 67 per cent in Lesotho. These results indicate that a large majority of those who have symptoms do seek treatment, though an appreciable minority do not. The small number of cases precluded any detailed examination of differentials. However, currently married men seek medical treatment more often than single men. Level of education also plays a positive role in willingness or ability to seek medical treatment.

In the Lusaka, Thailand and Rio de Janeiro surveys, respondents who reported at least one episode of STD infection in their lives were asked the following two questions: *On the last occasion when you had on STD, did you do anything to prevent your partner(s) (regular or casual) from getting this infection? Did you tell your partner that you had an STD?*

One possible response to the first question is that the respondent was infected by his partner. These respondents (small in number) have been excluded from the analysis. Responses indicate that a substantial proportion of men who ever had STDs claimed to have done something on the last occasion to prevent their partners from getting STDs. In Lusaka and Thailand 72 per cent did so and in Rio de Janeiro 56 per cent. There is no clear evidence of any strong associations between age, marital status, or education or media exposure and this form of preventive behaviour. Smaller proportions had told their partner that they had an STD. For those men who have had STDs, only 51 per cent in Lusaka and 49 per cent in Rio de Janeiro had informed their partner. In Thailand, such openness appears to be much less common; in this survey, only 17 per cent told their partner. Again, there is no appreciable effect of age of the respondent, marital status or education on the propensity to inform partners.

Knowledge of Protection against STDs

In a large number of surveys, knowledge of ways to prevent STDs was ascertained by the following question: *Do you know any ways in which you can avoid or protect yourself from getting these conditions? IF YES: what ways do you know?* This question was asked of all sexually active men. Sources of knowledge (e.g. doctors, friends, books) or effectiveness of the preventive methods were not assessed.

The proportion of respondents who reported that they knew at least one method to prevent STDs is highly variable across the countries surveyed: 35 per cent in Côte d'Ivoire; 43 per cent in Lesotho; 54 per cent in Tanzania;

65 per cent in Lusaka; 62 per cent in Manila; 94 per cent in Singapore; 85 per cent in Thailand; and 87 per cent in Rio de Janeiro. Moreover, these figures are difficult to interpret because of the vagueness of the question. In reality, nearly all respondents must have known that avoidance of certain types of sexual contact is one way to prevent STDs.

The level of declared knowledge is almost the same for all ages in the different countries. Education is the key determining factor. For instance, in Côte d'Ivoire, and among those who never attended school, only 12 per cent cited at least one way to prevent STDs as against 54 per cent for those who have secondary education. In Tanzania, the corresponding figures were 34 per cent versus 72 per cent; in Lusaka 41 per cent versus 70 per cent; and in Rio de Janeiro 73 per cent versus 95 per cent. It is reassuring to note that respondents who reported non-marital sexual contacts in the last 12 months were more likely to claim preventive knowledge than other respondents. Media exposure also seems to play a key role in the knowledge of a method to prevent STDs.

The nature and the safety of the methods of protection mentioned by the respondents were variable within and between populations. A large proportion of men reported that the method they know the best is the condom. Many others mentioned the avoidance of multiple partners and faithfulness to a regular partner. Taking antibiotics was another frequent answer, particularly in Côte d'Ivoire.

Drinking Habits

The optional section on alcohol was included in the survey protocol because alcohol use may be associated with risk taking and diminished self-control with regard to sexual behaviour. In addition to this effect of alcohol on mood and outlook, it is reasonable to expect a situational link between alcohol consumption and sexual behaviour. In many countries, commercial or other fleeting sexual contacts are made in bars and clubs that serve alcohol. Thus, simply on grounds of opportunity, a link between drinking and non-regular sex is plausible. The following surveys included this optional section of the questionnaire: Central African Republic, Côte d'Ivoire, Guinea-Bissau, Lesotho, Tanzania (KABP), Lusaka, Mauritius, Manila, Thailand and Rio de Janeiro.

An initial question was used as a relatively neutral introduction to the topic and to obtain an indication of the level of alcohol consumption. This question, however, may prove sensitive and embarrassing in societies where drinking alcoholic beverages is socially unacceptable and/or carries legal sanctions. In most of the societies studied this was not the case and no resistance to answering these questions was found. The relevant question was, *How often do you have drinks containing alcohol? Would you say: more than twice a week/Once or twice a week/Once or twice a month/Less often/Never.*

Table 7.3 provides estimates of all respondents who can be considered

Table 7.3: *Percentage of all respondents who drink alcohol once a week or more, by background characteristics*

Background Characteristics	CAR	Côte d'Ivoire	Guinea Bissau	Lesotho	Tanzania	Mauritius	Lusaka	Sri Lanka	Thailand	Rio de Janeiro
All	28.9	17.2	27.7	16.9	24.0	25.0	22.1	8.5	18.9	42.0
Male	37.0	24.8	31.4	27.5	29.2	43.5	37.7	15.7	38.5	57.4
Female	20.3	9.7	20.7	11.2	20.7	6.1	7.4	1.3	5.7	28.8
Age										
15–19	12.9	6.5	10.1	(3.7)	11.9	11.9	4.5	0.8	7.0	29.5
20–24	26.0	15.7	27.2	12.4	18.2	20.8	15.7	3.7	17.2	41.5
25–39	35.7	19.9	31.6	17.8	26.0	28.8	30.8	10.3	22.4	46.1
40–49	34.3	21.8	27.4	30.9	34.4	28.8	36.5	14.6	20.5	39.9
50+	31.7	28.2	33.3	20.7	33.6	25.9	26.8	–	–	–
Marital status										
Currently married	30.6	18.2	29.7	17.8	25.8	28.4	24.4	12.0	19.9	44.5
Formerly married	33.7	19.2	36.7	6.3	28.6	12.8	28.9	3.7	24.8	42.9
Never married	18.9	11.8	16.0	14.3	17.4	20.5	12.8	3.8	15.4	35.3
Education										
No school	25.4	17.4	22.6	30.1	21.7	19.8	13.0	–	17.2	35.5
Primary	29.6	16.8	24.2	16.5	25.1	29.6	17.1	–	19.3	42.6
Secondary+	34.1	17.3	37.7	12.5	23.4	21.5	26.5	–	18.2	45.5
Residence										
Urban	28.3	13.6	28.4	17.2	18.5	22.1	–	8.0	17.7	–
Rural	29.2	21.7	27.3	16.7	32.6	29.1	–	8.8	19.5	–
Risk behaviour										
No or limited risk	27.4	13.7	26.2	9.9	–	23.6	19.6	8.0	14.2	37.3
Some risk	42.4	29.2	30.9	28.7	–	54.0	42.1	60.6	54.8	71.2
Number	2431	3001	1297	1582	4084	2463	1992	3012	2801	1341

as regular alcohol consumers, drinking at least once a week. The prevalence of alcohol consumption is surprisingly uniform across these ten study populations. Sri Lanka and Rio de Janeiro are the outliers; only 9 per cent drink at least once a week in Sri Lanka compared to 42 per cent in Rio de Janeiro. In all other surveys, the proportions lie within the relatively narrow range of 17 to 29 per cent.

Differences between men and women are pronounced in all study populations, but particularly so in the Asian sites and in Mauritius, which, of course has a substantial population of Asian origin. Among the African surveys, there is considerable variability in the ratio of male to female drinkers; in Tanzania it is 1.4 to 1.0 while in Côte d'Ivoire and Lesotho it rises to 2.5 men to 1.0 women. There is no clear sub-regional pattern to these results.

In most surveys, drinking increases with age. The prevalence of alcohol consumption is invariably lowest among teenagers and usually lower among young adults age 20–24 years than among older persons. In Côte d'Ivoire and Sri Lanka, the proportions who drink continue to increase monotonically with age; but in other study populations, there is no clear-cut trend after the age of 25 years. Consistent with these results for age is an association with marital status. Single persons, most of whom are of course young, are less likely to drink than those who are currently married. In some sites, the highest level of drinking is found among the small formerly married category but this difference is by no means universal.

A positive link between education and alcohol consumption might have been anticipated because of the greater purchasing power of the better educated and their exposure to modern influences. However, the results in Table 7.3 reveal a variety of patterns. In Côte d'Ivoire, Tanzania, Thailand and Rio de Janeiro, there is essentially no difference across educational groups. In three other sites (Central African Republic, Guinea Bissau and Lusaka), those with secondary schooling are most likely to report regular drinking. In Lesotho, this relationship is reversed, while finally in Mauritius, the highest level of drinking is found among respondents with primary schooling.

Rural-urban differences in drinking habits can be assessed in five surveys. In three of these, the difference is small, leaving only Côte d'Ivoire and Guinea Bissau where the urban population is much more likely to drink regularly than those living in rural areas. Finally, a strong and consistent link between sexual risk behaviour and alcohol consumption is found. Respondents who reported non-marital sexual contacts in the last 12 months were typically 20 to 30 per cent more likely to be regular drinkers. This difference, however, is less pronounced in the cities of Rio de Janeiro and Lusaka.

Following the introductory question on regularity of drinking, respondents were asked a series of more focused questions. Those who had consumed alcohol in the last month were requested to recall the occasion (in the last few weeks) when they had drunk the most and were then asked how long they had spent drinking on that occasion. In most study populations, the majority had spent an hour or more drinking; the proportion lies between

80 and 90 per cent in Tanzania, Lusaka, Thailand and Rio de Janeiro. In Côte d'Ivoire, Guinea Bissau, and Manila, prolonged drinking appears to be less common; between 50 and 65 per cent gave answers of one hour or more. This proportion is lower still in Sri Lanka where only 37 per cent had spent at least one hour drinking.

Respondents were then asked, *Did you have sex on this occasion?* No distinction was made between regular and non-regular partners, thus the results are difficult to interpret with precision. However, cross-classification by marital status may reduce to some extent this ambiguity. As seen in Table 7.4, there is a remarkably strong link between drinking and sex, both for those who are married or in regular partnerships and those who are not. In five of eleven study populations, over one-fifth of unmarried persons reported the occurrence of sexual intercourse. By the definition used in these surveys, the partner must have been a sexual worker or non-regular associate. The exceptions are all non-African in character. Indeed, the only non-African population where there is a pronounced link between sex and alcohol for the unmarried is Thailand.

The proportion of currently married respondents who had sexual intercourse on this occasion of prolonged drinking is relatively similar in the African surveys to the proportion among the unmarried. We may only surmise that the sexual partner was often not the spouse. In contrast, among most of the non-African surveys, married persons were much more likely to report sex than the unmarried. For instance, in Sri Lanka, the difference is 36 versus 10 per cent and in Rio de Janeiro 23 versus 10 per cent.

In a smaller number of surveys, the link between alcohol and sex was pursued further by two rather different questions, one referring to meeting friends and sexual partners, and the other referring explicitly to casual sexual relations linked with alcohol consumption. The first formulation was used in Côte d'Ivoire, Guinea Bissau, Tanzania, Mauritius and Sri Lanka. The question was: *Do you think drinking helps you meet friends or sexual partners?* The second formulation was used in Lusaka, Manila, Thailand and Rio de Janeiro. The question was: *Do you usually have sex (with people other than your spouse/regular sex partner) when you have been drinking?* The results are summarized in Table 7.5 for respondents who drink at least once a week.

For these regular drinkers, only a limited proportion of 25 per cent or less reported that drinking helps them to meet friends or sex partners or that they regularly have sex after drinking. Those who have never been married were more likely to report that drinking can help, and there is a striking difference between those who report non-marital sex in the last 12 months and others. For instance 34 per cent of the former group compared to 14 per cent said that drinking helps to make friends or sexual partners. In Mauritius the corresponding percentages are 25 and 1 per cent. Men are much more likely than women to report that they usually have casual sex when they drink. There is also considerable consistency in the reporting of non-regular sex and answers to this latter question.

Table 7.4: *Among respondents who have had alcohol in the last four weeks, percentage who reported having had sex after longest drinking episode, by sex and marital status*

Background Characteristics	CAR	Côte D'Ivoire	Guinea Bissau	Lesotho	Tanzania	Lusaka	Mauritius	Manila	Sri Lanka	Thailand	Rio de Janeiro
All	40.4	30.2	17.5	42.2	18.5	25.1	9.4	14.3	31.0	33.5	19.4
Male	46.0	25.5	19.8	45.1	17.5	25.2	10.1	12.6	30.8	36.9	16.9
Female	29.5	42.1	10.9	38.5	19.6	24.2	4.1	19.0	33.3	18.8	23.6
Marital status											
Currently married	40.7	32.0	17.8	40.1	20.0	27.8	9.7	19.7	35.7	36.1	23.0
Formerly married	22.9	18.9	9.1	33.3	11.5	11.1	23.5	8.7	–	24.3	9.1
Never married	48.2	24.1	20.6	55.6	16.3	18.0	7.3	6.3	9.8	28.7	10.4
Number	697	517	354	254	768	395	616	530	242	519	562

Table 7.5: *Among respondents who have alcohol at least once a week, the percentage saying that (a) drinking helps to make friends/sexual partners; (b) they usually have non-marital sex after drinking*

Background Characteristics	(a) Friends or sexual partners						(b) Non-marital sex		
	CAR	Guinea Bissau	Tanzania	Mauritius	Sri Lanka	Lusaka	Manila	Thailand	Rio de Janeiro
All	23.1	13.9	24.2	3.4	15.0	14.4	7.0	23.8	12.6
Male	25.8	17.4	27.7	3.7	13.7	16.3	8.9	29.1	16.3
Female	13.0	4.5	21.1	1.4	35.7	5.5	2.9	0.0	6.3
Marital status									
Currently married	19.7	13.8	23.3	1.8	13.3	13.7	5.4	15.3	9.2
Formerly married	29.7	13.6	22.1	17.6	–	15.8	6.7	24.3	21.2
Never married	34.5	17.9	29.3	6.1	25.7	18.5	9.6	48.4	21.4
Risk behaviour									
No or limited risk	14.4	12.1	–	1.1	9.9	10.3	3.7	9.1	6.9
Some risk	33.7	17.6	–	24.6	70.0	29.2	28.9	52.8	31.3
Number	364	323	965	616	233	436	629	529	563

In conclusion, it appears that alcohol consumption is relatively common in most of the societies surveyed and that long sessions of drinking occur quite often, particularly among young adults. There is a strong relationship between alcohol consumption and sexual activity. The causal nature of this relationship, however, remains uncertain. Individuals may frequent bars and clubs where alcohol is served with the prime intention of finding a sexual partner. In such circumstances, alcohol consumption is part of the social setting for such encounters but not in itself necessarily a contributing factor. Conversely and perhaps more probably, alcohol consumption does indeed facilitate non-marital sex.

Medically Related Injection Practices

The section on injection practices was proposed because of the possible association between HIV infection and receipt of injections with shared and unsterilized needles. In many parts of the world, injections for medical reasons are preferred over oral medication and are often given outside the formal health care system, thus giving rise to concern about this mode of HIV transmission. Information was collected on respondent's experience with injections for medical reasons during the preceding 12 months. The question related to any type of injection, regardless of its purpose and the person who gave it. The following surveys included this section on injections: Central African Republic, Côte d'Ivoire, Guinea Bissau, Burundi, Tanzania (KABP), Lusaka, Mauritius, Manila, Thailand and Rio de Janeiro.

It is interesting to note from Table 7.6 that a very large proportion of the general population aged 15–49 years surveyed had received injections in the last 12 months: 55 per cent in the Central African Republic; between 40 and 50 per cent in Côte d'Ivoire, Guinea Bissau, Tanzania, Thailand and Rio de Janeiro; between 30 and 40 per cent in Burundi, Lusaka and Mauritius; but only 13 per cent in Manila. Generally, a slightly higher proportion of women report having received injections than men, but the incidence of medically related injections is approximately the same for all age groups. Higher educational achievement increases the probability of having received such injections, except in Mauritius and Thailand. Urban people receive more injections than those in the rural areas, with the exception of Mauritius and Thailand where this difference is reversed. In addition to the proportion of people receiving injections, the number of injections they received during the last year is also an important factor when considering the potential risk of HIV transmission. Accordingly, respondents were asked how many injections they had received in the last 12 months. For those who had received any injection in the last 12 months, the average number was between four and five for most of the countries, ranging from 3.0 in Manila; 3.8 in Côte d'Ivoire; to almost 5 in the Central African Republic, Guinea Bissau, Burundi, Lusaka, Thailand and Rio de Janeiro. It is apparent that, in most of these countries,

Table 7.6: Percentage of all respondents who had at least one injection in the last 12 months, by background characteristics

Background Characteristics	CAR	Côte d'Ivoire	Guinea Bissau	Burundi	Tanzania	Lusaka	Mauritius	Manila	Thailand	Rio de Janeiro
All	55.3	48.4	45.9	33.7	42.0	38.0	32.3	13.4	43.1	43.2
Male	50.2	46.1	44.9	25.4	36.2	35.9	34.0	11.0	38.1	43.0
Female	60.6	50.7	47.7	42.4	46.6	39.9	30.6	14.6	46.5	43.4
Age										
15–19	56.0	47.9	43.4	27.6	35.1	27.9	32.0	11.1	35.0	37.3
20–24	59.3	51.4	47.8	36.0	45.3	37.9	34.3	14.0	43.2	48.2
25–39	55.1	49.4	49.7	37.0	45.5	43.4	32.0	16.8	45.4	44.1
40–49	51.0	42.6	43.3	32.4	35.5	39.2	31.0	6.3	43.7	41.2
50+	49.5	45.7	40.8	–	40.0	33.9	32.7	13.9	–	–
Education										
No school	52.3	40.1	41.6	32.3	32.4	24.9	38.6	26.7	42.5	37.0
Primary	53.9	50.8	45.0	35.4	44.0	34.9	31.8	9.6	45.4	46.2
Secondary+	62.4	56.7	52.9	33.9	52.3	41.7	31.1	13.8	38.2	44.7
Residence										
Urban	63.7	51.6	52.0	35.7	48.4	–	28.8	–	36.9	–
Rural	50.8	44.5	42.3	31.8	33.1	–	37.3	–	46.1	–
Number	2318	3001	1297	2220	4171	1992	2463	1601	2801	1341
Mean number of injections (for those with 1+ injections)	4.8	3.8	5.6	5.0	4.2	5.2	–	3.0	4.6	4.8

nearly half of the population is receiving about five injections per year. Those who live in urban areas and those who are educated receive injections at a slightly higher rate than those who live in rural areas and those who have not attended school.

In conclusion, the absolute number of injections performed per year in these adult populations is more than twice the population size. Even with a very small proportion of HIV-infected needles, these high figures imply that the number of possible HIV transmissions through this route may be far from negligible.

Overview

Three main risk factors were analyzed in comparable general population surveys: STDs, alcohol consumption, and medically related injection practices. WHO/GPA surveys have provided much new information on these behavioural co-factors in HIV transmission.

STD prevention and treatment is now recognized to be an important component of sound HIV control programmes. The WHO/GPA surveys represent an important attempt to provide representative information on the incidence of STDs and/or symptoms. The results reported in this chapter reinforce the impression that STDs are a common occurrence in many populations and that prompt treatment is by no means universal. Indeed the situation may be worse than portrayed here, because of the likelihood of under-reporting. Validation of self-reported STDs is an urgent methodological priority.

We suspect that the WHO/GPA surveys have also furnished for some populations the first nationally representative data on alcohol consumption. A strong link between drinking and sexual behaviour that is of potential high risk emerges clearly. In Chapter 4, this link was confirmed statistically. Regular drinking was a predictor of the occurrence of non-marital sex, after controlling for many of the obvious confounding factors. The results here tend to confirm anecdotal and observational evidence that, in many societies, episodes of casual sex start in bars, clubs and dance halls where alcohol consumption is an intrinsic part of the proceedings. The obvious policy response is to ensure that condoms are readily available at such places. A more imaginative strategy is to enlist bar men, club owners and other staff as promoters of safe sex. A number of such schemes have now been tried.

With regard to injections, WHO/GPA surveys can only demonstrate the vast number of medically related injections that occur each year in most societies. Even if a small proportion of needles are shared, the potential risk of HIV transmission would be very great. Perhaps renewed emphasis should be given to the need for sterilized or disposable needles, particular in countries where many injections occur outside the formal health sector and are given by unqualified practitioners.

Chapter 8

Summary and Conclusions

John Cleland with Benoît Ferry and Michel Caraël

Principal Findings

Results presented in the previous chapters come from nine sites in continental sub-Saharan Africa, four in Asia and two from elsewhere. Twelve of these samples had national coverage while the remaining three were restricted to capital cities. Clearly this distribution of research locations prevents any generalization of results to developing countries as a whole and severely curtails inter-regional comparison. On the other hand, the relatively good representation of sites in sub-Saharan Africa may permit the drawing of tentative conclusions at a regional level.

The limitations of geographical coverage should not blind us to the magnitude of new evidence represented by these surveys. Previously, no national surveys on sexual behaviour had ever been undertaken in developing countries, and surveys on AIDS-related knowledge and attitudes were sparse in number. Only in regard to condom knowledge and use did the WHO/GPA programme follow in the pathway of others, although even here the information gathered from men, as well as from women, is largely new. The research findings reported in this volume therefore cannot be judged by their contribution to a pre-existing body of knowledge. Rather, they represent the start of a new domain of scientific information on a hitherto neglected topic. This contribution of new information is particularly marked with regard to sexual behaviour itself. We start this overview, therefore, by outlining what has been learnt about behaviour, before proceeding to discuss results on cognitive and attitudinal dimensions.

Sexual Behaviour

Chapter 4 covers a wide terrain though it should be noted that the topics of bisexuality and homosexuality were not covered in most surveys. The onset of heterosexual activity and patterns of sexual behaviour before the first marriage are discussed. Regular partnerships are analyzed in terms of polygamy, cohabitation, coital frequency; finally results on relationships with non-regular partners and with sex workers are presented. Some of these topics are not entirely new for survey research. Information on age at first intercourse is routinely collected in the Demographic and Health Surveys (DHS) project which has sponsored national surveys in over 30 developing countries (Blanc and Rutenberg, 1990). Marriage, naturally, has been widely studied, though usually with a somewhat narrower definition than the one used in the WHO/GPA surveys. However, information on sexual relationships outside of stable partnerships has never previously been collected through national surveys, and it is on this aspect that we now wish to concentrate.

The reason for the attention given by WHO/GPA to what we shall loosely term non-marital sex is obvious. Of all the risk factors for sexually transmitted disease, including HIV, the number of recent sexual partners has proved, in epidemiological research, to be consistently one of the most important, at least in contexts where unprotected sex is widely practised (Anderson, 1992). Measurement of the numbers of partners, particularly those of a non-regular nature, was thus a high priority, because of the potential importance of this factor in HIV transmission. The word *potential* should be stressed. Clearly, the actual risk of infection to individuals depends on the overall prevalence of HIV in their particular communities and networks, as well as on condom use. The research sites represented in this volume varied greatly in this regard. In some sites, the virus had spread widely among the general population by the late 1980s. In such settings, almost any unprotected act of intercourse outside mutually faithful partnerships represented some risk of HIV infection, and infection via the spouse was an additional hazard. In others, HIV/AIDS was almost entirely absent and thus a rapid rate of partner change did not imply any appreciable risk of infection. When the prevalence of HIV infection becomes very high, the number of partners also becomes a less important risk factor. Thus there should be no implication that identical behaviours carry the same health risk in different locations.

What picture emerges from the surveys of sexual behaviour outside marriage that carries an actual or potential future risk of HIV infection? For ease of reference, some key results are summarized in Table 8.1. There are several striking features. First, there is a huge difference between men and women in reported behaviour. Men are much more likely to report non-marital sexual contacts in the past 12 months than women, and the contrast is particularly pronounced among the non-African surveys. This difference has been found in all sexual behaviour surveys to date and has generated much discussion. Differential reporting by men and women, differences in perceptions of what constitutes a regular as opposed to a non-regular partner, and probable omission from the sampling frames of female sex workers are most plausible reasons for the discrepancy. The analysis in Chapter 4 suggests that sex involving payment – likely to be reported by many male clients but by few, if any, female sex workers – is probably not the main explanation. Even when those reporting sex in exchange for money, gifts or favours are removed, there still remains a wide gulf between what men and

Table 8.1: Key behavioural indicators

Surveys	Percentage of all respondents reporting non-regular sex in last 12 months		Percentage of all men reporting 5 or more non-regular partners in last 12 months	Among men who reported commercial sex in last 12 months, percentage who always used condoms on these occasions
	Men	Women	Men	Men
CAR	13.6	4.7	1.6	18.4
Côte d'Ivoire	50.7	13.4	9.7	11.4
Guinea Bissau	43.5	20.5	0.6	na
Togo	19.5	1.3	1.7	7.7
Burundi	7.1	1.9	1.5	25.6
Kenya	30.9	12.2	4.1	na
Lesotho	23.7	19.1	7.7	15.1
Tanzania	32.0	14.0	5.1	8.4
Lusaka	35.9	9.7	7.8	24.7
Mauritius	9.9	0.2	na	na
Manila	14.9	1.2	1.2	20.6
Singapore	9.8	0.6	3.2	27.6
Sri Lanka	4.3	3.1	0.4	na
Thailand	28.2	1.7	11.2	33.1
Rio de Janeiro	44.3	9.8	10.2	5.0

na = Not available

what women say. Similarly, there is little support for the thesis that women are more likely than men to portray sexual partners as *regular* on a scale sufficient to explain the divide. We are left then with the probability of differential reporting that, given the relatively short recall period, must be more a reflection of conscious misreporting than memory lapse. Might men overreport sexual contacts outside marriage or regular partnerships? It is certainly a possibility, but two strands of evidence suggest, obliquely, that this may not be the case. First, the assessment of inter-partner consistency in the reporting of coital frequency does not reveal any systematic exaggeration by men (see Chapter 2). And second, there is a remarkable consistency in men's and women's reporting of multiple regular partnerships (see Figure 4.10), which suggests that men do not inflate this dimension of their lives. These results fall a long way short of proving that men do not overreport their numbers of non-regular partners, but they are at least suggestive that this type of respondent error may not be common. By this process of elimination, there remains the possibility that women are more likely to underreport 'non-marital' relationships than men. This factor, we suggest, is likely to be a particularly important, though not the only, reason for the substantial gender difference in the reporting of non-marital sex. This very tentative conclusion warns us against naïve, literal interpretation of survey results.

The second striking feature of the results on non-marital sex is the fact that, with only one marginal exception, a substantial proportion of individuals in each study site reported no sexual contact outside regular partnerships in the last 12 months. Restricting attention to men for reasons outlined above, there is, however, considerable inter-survey variability, ranging from over 40 per cent reporting at least one contact to less than 5 per cent. Some features of this variability are consistent with prior knowledge of the cultures involved. For instance, it is not perhaps surprising that the reported prevalence of non-marital sex is low in Sri Lanka, Singapore and Mauritius, all societies characterized by restrictive sexual values, but much higher in Thailand, Rio de Janeiro and most of the African sites. In other regards, inter-survey differences have no immediate explanation and only further study, including repeated surveys, will show whether they are genuine or artifacts of differential reporting. For instance, the small proportion of men in Burundi, a country with a relatively high level of HIV, who report non-regular sex is surprising.

To return to the key point, the majority of men in all sites reported no sexual associates outside of regular partnerships in the year preceding the survey. Furthermore, the proportions claiming five or more such associates are consistently low, ranging from zero to 12 per cent. These results are totally incompatible with the view, prevalent only a few years ago, that the HIV pandemic in Africa was fuelled by extreme promiscuity. For instance, when a group of experts met in 1990 to assess different mathematical models for projecting the spread of HIV by standardizing the input parameters, the behavioural assumptions included one that men, on average, have 12 sexual partners per year (UN/WHO, 1991). The WHO/GPA surveys suggest that a value closer to two would have been more realistic. Of course the survey estimates might be too low even for men because of underreporting, but it would be unreasonable to suppose that this factor could bridge the difference between about 2 and 12 partners per year.

WHO/GPA surveys are thus immensely valuable in correcting wildly inaccurate perceptions of sexual behaviour, that were based on guesswork or small unrepresentative studies. They have also helped to destroy stereotypes about sexual behaviour in Africa. The results from the African surveys do not portray a region with uniquely high levels of partner change. The results from Thailand and Rio de Janeiro, for instance, are not so different, nor are some of those recently obtained in Europe (ACSF Investigators, 1992; Johnson, *et al.* 1992; Spira, Bajos and Groupe ACSF, 1993).

The behavioural data furnished by the WHO/GPA programme, represent a huge potential improvement in the empirical foundations of mathematical models of HIV transmission and demonstrate the inadequacy of our current understanding of the epidemiology of the disease. The political impact of the findings may prove to be equally valuable in undermining dangerous, even racist, stereotypes of different cultures. Finally, the survey results provide a basis for cautious optimism on the grounds that, for much of the time, substantial proportions of men and women may confine sexual activity to regular partnerships and therefore are not at high risk of infection. While we cannot draw definite conclusions about overall sexual lifestyles, because detailed information was collected only for the most recent 12 month period, nevertheless it is valid to conclude that non-marital sex is a relatively rare event for a majority of men and women.

PR, and to a lesser extent KABP, surveys allow us not only to describe the prevalence at the national level of certain types of sexual relationship that have implications for HIV/AIDS, but to examine how these behaviours vary between demographic and socio-economic strata. In broad terms, the prevalence of sexual contacts outside regular partnerships (if any) is most common among young adults aged in their early twenties, and more common among the single than the married. Typically, the occurrence of non-marital contacts declines after the age of 25 years.

Educational attainment is positively associated with the prevalence of non-marital sex, though not in all study populations. The reason for this link may reflect the higher incomes of the better educated, as much as any direct influence of schooling on sexual values and attitudes. More surprisingly, there was little support for the commonsense assumption that towns and cities are more conducive to the formation of non-regular sexual relationships than rural areas. After controls for education, marital status and other factors, urban–rural differences were weak and inconsistent. Sexual behaviour in rural and urban areas of the same country were strongly correlated, thus further emphasizing that the transition from a rural to an urban environment does not mark any major discontinuity in sexual outlook or opportunity. It may also be noted that regular alcohol consumption was strongly associated with non-marital sex, though causal interpretation of this relationship is not straightforward.

Perhaps more fascinating than an examination of the relationships between individual characteristics and sexual behaviour is the identification of different sexual regimes at the societal level. The evidence from these 16 surveys suggests that there is a strong link between the prevalence of virginity at first marriage for women and the lack of extra-marital contacts among women. The degree of social control on the premarital sexual behaviour of women appears to be strongly correlated with the degree of control after marriage. However, restrictive norms for women do not imply similar restrictions for men. At the societal level, there was no association between the prevalence of virginity at marriage for women and men. Nor was the level of female virginity associated with the prevalence of non-regular or commercial sex among men. Finally, there is a suggestion that societies where multiple and non-cohabiting regular partnerships are relatively common may be characterized by high levels of sexual contact outside regular partnerships. The pattern, like others, is based on findings from only 16 data sets and thus should be advanced with considerable caution but it indicates that the predominant characteristics of marital or regular partnerships may condition non-marital sexual behaviour. The nature of these partnerships reflects to some extent, the structure of economics. In many countries, an increasingly difficult search for employment results in long-term spousal separations. Thus,

Table 8.2: Key indicators of knowledge, beliefs and attitudes

Survey	Percentage of all respondents aware of AIDS	Among respondents aware of AIDS, percentage believing that touching someone with AIDS can transmit infection	Percentage of all men aware of condoms and source of supply	Among respondents aware of AIDS, percentage reporting themselves to be at moderate or high risk of HIV infection
CAR	83	60	43	60
Côte d'Ivoire	90	51	46	37
Guinea Bissau	75	69	31	30
Togo	64	40	48	27
Burundi	96	77	48	6
Kenya	89	75	54	13
Lesotho	98	67	67	8
Tanzania	96	66	na	5
Lusaka	98	88	60	10
Mauritius	92	49	79	3
Manila	98	76	64	5
Singapore	95	79	93	0
Sri Lanka	77	39	na	2
Thailand	99	63	89	19
Rio de Janeiro	100	93	85	9

na = Not available

a complete interpretation of sexual behaviour has to take into account the economic structure.

We end this brief overview of behavioural findings with the sobering data on condom use for sexual contacts that involved the exchange of money, gifts or favours. Those relationships do not necessarily involve professional sex workers, but nevertheless represent sexual behaviour that carries a relatively high actual or potential risk of HIV infection. As shown in Table 8.1, the percentage of men who consistently used condoms in these situations ranges from only about 5 to 30 per cent. These results demonstrate vividly the magnitude of the task ahead for HIV-prevention programmes.

Cognitive and Attitudinal Dimensions

In this section, we outline some of the key results that have been presented on knowledge, beliefs and attitudes concerning HIV/AIDS (Chapter 3), condoms (Chapter 5) and perceived risk and behavioural change (Chapter 6). It may appear illogical to discuss behavioural change here rather than in the previous section but, as will be argued, the results on this topic reveal more about attitudes than about actual modifications in overt sexual behaviour. As before, a few major indicators are shown for ease of reference (Table 8.2).

Before discussing the results themselves, it should be recalled that most of the surveys were conducted in 1989 or 1990. Unlike behaviour itself (in most circumstances), knowledge can change very rapidly and it should be borne in mind, therefore, that the climate of knowledge and outlook in the populations surveyed may now be very different.

Despite this caveat, it is clear that an awareness of HIV/AIDS was already very widespread in all the study populations by the late 1980s, even in those settings where the disease was not a serious public health concern. Moreover, knowledge of sexual transmission of HIV was also very high. Such 'correct' knowledge, however, co-exists with beliefs in modes of transmission that have no scientific justification. Touching people with AIDS, sharing their cooking utensils, or wearing their clothes were all endorsed by substantial proportions (in many instance, by over 50 per cent) as potential routes of transmission. These misfounded beliefs cannot be attributed to general ignorance or isolation from sources of information. They are as common in Rio de Janeiro and Singapore, for instance, as among the least educated of the study populations. They also remain widespread in some industrialized countries (e.g. Dab *et al.*, 1989; Moatti, 1992). Clearly, then, continuing belief in casual modes of transmission are not easily dislodged by public information campaigns. Perhaps individuals find it difficult to accept that HIV is so different from other much more infectious diseases. A further contributing factor is that some of these modes of transmission were discredited only recently by medical scientists.

The majority of respondents in nearly all study sites was aware of the seriousness of HIV/AIDS. Typically, between 65 to 85 per cent thought that all or most persons with AIDS will die of this condition. Similarly, only minorities, ranging from 3 to 30 per cent, thought that AIDS is curable. Accurate knowledge of the consequences of HIV is thus widespread but by no means universal. There remain appreciable minorities who possess optimistic views. This appreciation of the consequences of HIV infection for individuals is paralleled by an awareness of its threat at the global and national level. Even in societies where very few AIDS cases had been reported, there was no widespread denial of the risk. Moreover, in most sites, the risk was perceived to be increasing.

The emphatic nature of these survey results on HIV/AIDS knowledge and attitude comes as a surprise. A common accusation is that governments and communities have been slow to recognize the seriousness of the situation and prone to deny the need for urgent, preventive action. Such denial has not been found among ordinary citizens. On the contrary, most recognize the essential, dangerous characteristics of HIV/AIDS and accept it as a top priority public health issue.

As greater use of condoms is one of the main ways of checking HIV, knowledge of and attitudes towards condoms were investigated in considerable detail in most PR and KABP surveys. Huge variations in condom awareness were apparent. In some sites, almost everyone had at least heard of condoms, whereas in others over half were completely ignorant. The lowest levels of knowledge were found in Africa, though within this region, knowledge varied greatly between populations.

Awareness of the method is not the only logical precondition for its use. Knowledge of a nearby source of supply is an equally powerful precondition and, in most WHO/GPA surveys, relevant information was obtained. The results in Table 8.2 speak for themselves. In five of the African sites, less than half of men and women were aware of condoms *and* knew where they could be obtained. When the additional criterion of reasonable access is added, in terms of living or working within 30 minutes of a source, the picture that emerges for Africa is even more depressing. In most of the African surveys, only a small minority of persons were classified as possessing sufficient knowledge and access for condom use. In the late 1980s, the huge task of creating the conditions where condom use would be at least a feasible option had hardly begun.

As is well known in family planning and health research, knowledge and access are not the sole, or even perhaps the critical, determinants of use. Perceived need to use condoms, beliefs in their effectiveness, harmlessness, ease of use, affordability and inoffensiveness to partners are among the many factors that may act in isolation or concert to promote or prevent condom use for pregnancy and disease prevention. Clearly some of these factors require sensitive, in-depth research for proper elucidation and, ultimately, quasi-experimental approaches may be required to assess whether these and other barriers to more widespread use of condoms can be overcome. Nevertheless, large scale standardized surveys provide a unique opportunity for describing the climate of public opinion about condoms, even if they cannot measure the relative importance of these opinions as influences on use.

The popular image of condoms that emerges from WHO/GPA surveys is surprisingly favourable. The majority of men and women accept that it is an effective method, both for pregnancy and STD prevention. Price is not viewed as a problem nor is difficulty of use, though, understandably, those who have never tried condoms tend to be unsure. Opposition based on religious beliefs is confined to a minority in most study populations. On the negative side, condoms are likely to be regarded as detrimental to sexual pleasure and a worryingly large minority in many surveys see a potential health hazard, by endorsing the belief that condoms may enter the womb or stomach of women.

As mentioned in Chapter 5, condoms have been associated historically with illicit sex and have not proved popular as a routine method of marital family planning. This attribute of condoms is clearly evident in the survey findings. They are much more likely to be seen as appropriate for sexual encounters outside of marriage than within marriage. Averaged across all surveys, nearly 40 per cent of men and women regard their use as offensive to a spouse. The social image of condoms is clearly one potential obstacle to wider use.

Taken at face value, these opinions on condoms give a relatively

favourable prognosis for increased condom use for intermittent or commercial sex relationships, but provide less grounds for optimism regarding condom use within more stable partnerships. Some further strands of evidence
support this interpretation; others, however, do not. There is clearly a link
between the occurrence of non-marital sex and condom use. As shown in
Chapter 5, respondents who reported non-regular sexual contacts in the last
12 months were much more likely to have used condoms, even after adjustment for other predictors. However, it is apparent from the analysis in Chapter 6 that greater use of condoms is rarely mentioned as a behavioural response
to the threat of HIV, nor do men who regularly use condoms during encounters with sex workers appear to gain any benefit in terms of perceived reduction in the risk of HIV infection.

The WHO/GPA surveys are thus giving complex, and somewhat contra-
dictory, messages about prospects for greater use of condoms. But the
overridingly important result is that rather few people in Africa could use
condoms if they wished, because of lack of effective access.

Earlier in this Chapter we have noted the fact that a majority of men and
women do not report sexual behaviour that might enhance the risk of HIV
infection. It might reasonably be inferred that a similar, or even larger,
majority would deny therefore any personal vulnerability or risk of HIV infection, except perhaps in settings where overall infection levels were very
high. This inference is not confirmed. In nine of the 15 study populations,
well over half of men and women thought themselves to be at some risk of
HIV infection, or were unsure of the risks. Thus, instead of attempting to
explain why denial of personal risk is so common, we are in the unexpected
position of having to account for a remarkably high level of perceived risk,
particularly among the African sites.

Reported sexual behaviour itself is not a major determinant of a sense
of vulnerability; persons who report no sexual activity at all in the preceding
12 months are almost as likely to feel themselves at some risk of HIV infection as those who reported contacts with non-regular partners or with sex
workers. Fear of infection by a spouse or regular partner may be part of the
explanation; in particular, it may help to account for the fact that women
feel as personally vulnerable as men. Belief in casual transmission is another
possible explanation. As shown earlier, such beliefs are very common. However, at the individual level, a belief in the possibility of infection through
touching a person with AIDS or by other casual routes did not emerge as a
significant predictor of personal risk. The wide, rather diffuse sense of vulnerability, that appears to have little rational basis in behaviour, thus remains
rather a mystery.

Of all the topics covered in KABP and PR surveys, behavioural change
is the most important, but has also proved the most intractable. Respondents
were asked whether they had modified their behaviour in response to the
threat of AIDS and, if so, in what main way. In all the African surveys, and
in Thailand and Rio de Janeiro, over 50 per cent of men report behavioural

change, typically by a reduction in non-regular partners or in their use of sex workers. Understandably, women are less likely to report this type of change. For reasons that are elaborated in Chapter 6, those results give an unduly optimistic picture; it is most unlikely that changes in behaviour have occurred on the scale suggested by those verbal testimonies. Nevertheless, the results are encouraging; the climate of opinion appears to be favourable to the idea of behavioural change. The prognosis would be much more pessimistic had the surveys found evidence of widespread denial of risk and unwillingness to contemplate the need for change.

As mentioned earlier, greater use of condoms was mentioned only rarely as a behavioural response to AIDS. However, it is likely that the phrasing of the relevant question with its emphasis on behaviour, steered respondents towards answering in terms of choice and number of partners and away from mentioning condom use. Certainly there is evidence of increased condom use for some countries. In Thailand, for instance, distributions and sales of condoms rose from 10 million in 1989 to over 100 million pieces in 1991. As the condom is not a common method of birth control, it is reasonable to infer that disease control is the predominant motive driving this huge increase.

Key Policy Implications

KABP, and a lesser extent, PR surveys were designed primarily to guide the National AIDS Control Programmes that were initiated in many countries in the late 1980s. The intention in this section is not to document the utility of survey results for specific national settings but rather to outline their strategic implications and general lessons for policies and programmes.

Descriptive surveys of general populations are often criticized for their lack of programme relevance. Indeed it is true that such surveys rarely give direct guidance on issues such as the appropriateness or relative cost-effectiveness of different interventions or public information campaigns. For this purpose, more focused operational research is needed. Nevertheless, the broad background information derived from surveys on people's sexual lives, their use of, and access to condoms, their knowledge of and fears about HIV/AIDS is of immense value. To reiterate a point made earlier, our ignorance of these topics in most developing countries was almost total at the time the surveys reported here were conducted and there was a real danger that AIDS prevention activities would be based on wildly erroneous assumptions.

By furnishing an abundance of detailed numerical information, WHO/ GPA and other similar surveys have helped to define the contours of the problem. The claim is not that survey results are infallibly true. This is far from the case. But numerical results, based on reasonably representative samples, inevitably stimulate debate and reaction during which new perceptions and directions may emerge. In the context of HIV/AIDS they also direct our attention to the lives of ordinary men and women, whose behaviour will ultimately decide the future course of the pandemic. This more socio-cultural perspective is surely an indispensable complement to bio-medical approaches. As will be argued later in this chapter, the value of surveys becomes even greater when they are repeated at regular intervals and thus can monitor progress towards desired goals.

From these generalities, we turn to the more specific strategic implications of the survey results. Perhaps the most important is the encouragement given to governments and other institutions to place HIV/AIDS prevention high on the agenda. People are concerned about HIV/AIDS; they recognize it as a growing international and national problem; many of them see it as a more personal threat; and they appear to offer little resistance to the idea of behavioural change. There is nothing in the survey findings to suggest that information about AIDS will be found offensive, irrelevant or counter-productive.

In terms of information needs, the task of spreading basic awareness is probably almost accomplished by now and there also appears little need to inform people about sexual transmission. However, beliefs in casual modes of transmission are prevalent. This is clearly an area that deserves attention because misinformation of this type might lend to a sense of helplessness and to discrimination against people thought to be HIV positive.

The dangers of discrimination are reinforced by other survey results. Restrictive, or even punitive, measures to check the disease were frequently advocated by survey respondents. Thus far, most countries have done re-markably well in combating prejudice and stigma, following the lead of WHO/GPA and other international organizations. This effort must be maintained not only for humanitarian reasons but also because of the practical consideration that fear of hostility will drive the disease underground and inhibit people from being tested and counselled.

Very few research teams chose to incorporate questions on sexual attitudes and therefore the surveys can offer little guidance on the content or credibility of messages about sexual conduct itself. However, the results attest to a widespread receptivity to exhortations about safer sex, as evidenced by the remarkably high proportions who claim that they have already curtailed sexual activities in response to the AIDS threat.

On condom promotion, more detailed findings are available. Here, the main practical value has been to document the totally inadequate levels of knowledge and access in much of Africa. While attitudes towards condoms appear surprisingly favourable, the majority of men and women simply do not have adequate access for purchase and use. Lack of knowledge can be overcome relatively easily by extensive publicity; the main constraint is likely to be lack of political will rather than money. Lack of access is obviously more problematic. By suggesting that price is not widely perceived as a deterrent to use, the surveys provide indirect support for greatly increased social marketing of condoms. However, the ability and willingness of individuals to pay should be assessed more rigorously than is possible from a single cross-sectional survey. Pricing policies are of huge practical importance and therefore justify careful experimental work.

Condom use is clearly associated in the minds of many people with non-marital sex and encounters with sex workers. Obviously, one priority of HIV prevention campaigns is to encourage condom use in such situations. In the late 1980s, regular condom use in relationships with sex workers was the exception rather than the norm in all study populations. Moreover, only minorities believed that condoms were effective against transmission of HIV. This scepticism, which contrasts with much more widespread acceptance of the efficacy of condoms against other sexually transmitted diseases, may reflect the persistence of beliefs in the casual transmission of HIV. In the public mind, contagiousness and lethality are perhaps difficult to disentangle. Whatever the reason, there is a strong case for enhancing awareness of the protective value of condoms.

There is a real dilemma here for public information campaigns. Certainly, condom use has to be promoted in circumstances where the serostatus of the partner is unknown, such as may be the case in transitory sex encounters, or relationships with sex workers. But these messages may reinforce an identification of condoms with illicit sex that already exists, and thereby indirectly discourage use within more enduring relationships. Once HIV has spread widely among the heterosexual population, condom use within marriage becomes an urgent necessity. The difficult challenge ahead is to raise drastically levels of condom use in potentially high risk ephemeral sexual contacts, without diminishing the chance that they will be used, when appropriate, in other circumstances.

The surveys provide little encouragement for attempts to raise further a sense of public danger and personal risk about AIDS. As noted earlier, surprisingly large numbers of people already feel at some risk of infection, often with apparently little justification. The sense of vulnerability is only weakly related to behaviour. It is of concern to note that, even among men who report five or more non-marital partners in the last 12 months, a substantial proportion, ranging from 20 to 50 per cent, perceive no risk of HIV infection to themselves. Condom use is not the explanation for this perception; it is rather low, as we have already seen. Similarly, it is of concern that so many monogamous individuals feel at risk, perhaps because of beliefs in casual transmission or fears of future unfaithfulness by their partner. One possible aim of public information campaigns might be to strengthen the link, in people's minds, between behaviour and risk; instilling more realistic perceptions would involve reassuring those in mutually lifelong monogamous relationships that they have little to fear, but also impressing upon others that they are putting themselves, and perhaps their regular partners, at risk.

The survey data on sexual behaviour itself contain several important policy messages. First, the majority of women and approximately two-thirds of men profess faithfulness to their regular partners. Maintenance of such behaviours for women is thus as important as attempts to curtail or modify men's non-marital sexual relationships. As stated earlier, these survey results, if valid, provide grounds for optimism; the behaviour of the majority is not conducive to further, rapid increases in HIV incidence and prevalence.

In terms of identifying specific priority groups for interventions and focused information campaigns, the analysis has made only a modest contribution. Rather, the lesson is that national programmes need to direct attention to the general population, and particularly to men. One clear message is the need to address the reproductive health needs of the very young in certain societies. There is sometimes a tendency to ignore persons aged less than 15 years in discussions of HIV prevention. Yet, the survey data show that by this age a large proportion are already sexually active. This is particularly true of Africa, where between 20 and 50 per cent of 15 year olds report sexual experience. Moreover, many sexually active teenagers report multiple partners, and condom use also tends to be low. Regardless of political or religious opposition, it is essential that safer sex education (knowledge of reproductive health, decision-making skills, negotiation skills and principles of safer sex) be taught to girls and boys in their early teens.

The surveys also warn against neglect of the rural population. While it is true that HIV prevalence is often much higher in major cities than elsewhere, the behaviours that underline HIV transmission are not so different. And finally it would be wrong to assume that the better educated are able to protect themselves against HIV and other sexually transmitted diseases. While condom use is certainly higher among the better educated, so too is non-marital sex.

Methodological Lessons

Before identifying the methodological lessons learned from the WHO/GPA sponsored KABP and PR surveys, it is appropriate to reflect for a moment on their origins and some of their more obvious achievements. As the magnitude of the HIV pandemic became apparent in the 1980s and funding for research was mobilized in response, social scientists in WHO/GPA might well have focused research exclusively on behaviours that appeared to be particularly implicated in HIV transmission: injecting drug use, sex work, homosexuality and bisexuality. Indeed coordinated programmes of research in all these specialist areas were initiated by WHO/GPA.

However, an early commitment was also made to the investigation of sexual behaviour, and HIV-relevant knowledge and beliefs, among general populations. This decision was forward looking, required courage and incurred an element of risk. The decision was forward looking because it recognized that, while the early phase of the epidemic in any country might be restricted to persons with clearly identifiable high risk behaviours, sooner or later, infection was likely to spread more widely unless rapid behavioural change occurred. This diffusion has already happened in some African countries and is now occurring elsewhere in South and Central America, the Caribbean and Asia. In many countries, where heterosexual transmission was not predominant from the start, it has become increasingly common as the epidemic matures. HIV prevention is thus a problem for entire societies and not merely for special groups. WHO/GPA's research priorities reflected this judgement.

The decision required courage because, hitherto, very few studies had been conducted of sexual behaviour among general populations. Moreover, most such studies were North American and were restricted to sexual behaviour within marriage. As noted earlier in this volume, the idea of conducting sex surveys among representative samples in many countries was initially greeted with incredulity or derision. Respondents would refuse to participate, it was claimed, or provide totally unreliable information. One of the achievements of the WHO/GPA programme of survey research has been to demonstrate that such surveys can be conducted successfully in many – perhaps most – developing countries without causing outrage or offence, at least within the context of a major pandemic involving a sexually transmissible agent. Refusal rates were generally low. It is the consensus now among WHO/GPA national investigators that surveys on sex are little different from surveys on more anodyne topics, and problems faced in the field are often concerned with how to conduct good surveys rather than how to conduct surveys on sex. Certainly, sensitivity is needed in approaching communities and the development of trust and rapport between interviewer and respondent is vital. But in most other practical aspects these surveys encountered no more problems than demographic or other types of enquiry. Similar conclusions have been reached with regard to sex surveys in industrialized countries (e.g. ACSF, 1992; Johnson, 1992).

As often happens, the main opposition at country level came from people with educated, middle-class backgrounds, including government officials and researchers themselves. WHO/GPA devoted considerable energy and ingenuity to overcoming these misgivings where they arose. A total of four regional and many other meetings were held to introduce, and justify the need for, KABP and PR surveys, and developing country academics were invited to play an active role in protocol development. The reputation of WHO was crucial to the success of this exercise. Probably no other institution could have persuaded so many government ministries to give their blessing to large scale surveys on sexual behaviour, or so many academics to devote their time and stake their reputations on a new and controversial domain of enquiry. The success of WHO in this regard will be of lasting benefit. Now that the taboo on sexual behaviour research has been largely broken, it is most unlikely to be recreated. Whatever the particular shortcomings of WHO/GPA's research programme, it has paved the way for future studies.

A further notable achievement of the WHO/GPA programme was the comprehensive nature of its recommendations on survey design and implementation. Most centrally coordinated cross-cultural research studies produce detailed data collection instruments or schedules but little other documentation. WHO/GPA went far beyond the norm. Its research package for PR surveys, for instance, contains a draft questionnaire, study design, a draft interviewer's manual, instructions for data entry and editing, recommendations for variable construction and a detailed tabulation plan. Even SPSS™ commands for variable creation and tabulation were issued. Rarely have such complete and detailed manuals of instructions been produced and this legacy of the exercise should also have an enduring value in guiding future researchers.

Perhaps because of the very detailed protocols produced at WHO/GPA headquarters, direct technical assistance to investigators was modest and in some instances inadequate. There was nearly always an in-country visit made by a WHO/GPA staff member or consultant to discuss overall design, but thereafter research teams were left largely to their own devices, with only perhaps one further visit to assist in data management. This arrangement often worked well and was clearly in the interests of fostering national research capacity and a sense of local ownership of the survey. But there were also occasions when more in-country guidance was needed. This is specially true with sample design, at the very start, and, again towards the end, with data management. As mentioned in Chapter 2, most of the principal investigators were senior social scientists or medical officers, often with a close involvement with the National AIDS Control Programme. While their research backgrounds were impressive, very few had prior experience of designing a nationally representative sample. Indeed this experience is often confined to staff of national statistical offices who have the mandate to conduct such surveys on a wide variety of topics. Of course, investigators were advised to consult their respective statistical offices about sample design and most did so. Regrettably, the final outcome was not always satisfactory. As documented in Chapter 2, the compositions of a few national surveys have an unmistakable urban bias that undermines claims to representativeness.

With regard to data management, defects were less far reaching in their implications. At worst, a few variables were lost because of inadequate data entry. More commonly, delays in producing results were experienced and files received at WHO headquarters required considerable further editing and documentation.

From these general considerations we turn now to an assessment of the substance of WHO/GPA surveys. In deciding topics for inclusion and measurement issues there was little prior experience to act as a guide. Objectives were broadly defined and the approach, while drawing upon the theoretical literature, was essentially descriptive. Decisions were reached, after numerous iterations, by groups and committees. Such a combination can be a recipe for disaster. Research instruments that arise from these circumstances typically lack focus and cultural specificity; by accommodating many views, offence may be minimized, but at the cost of failing to address any particular topic in sufficient depth or detail. Moreover, any programme of standardized cross-cultural survey research is prone to inflexibility. Lessons learnt in the early studies can only be incorporated into later studies at the expense of comparability. There is thus a strong temptation to resist the introduction of improvements, and progress towards better designs is thereby stifled.

This pessimistic picture is not intended as criticism of WHO/GPA's efforts. The features enumerated above are almost inevitable consequences of centrally coordinated cross-cultural research. Nor is any apology needed for the descriptive rather than theoretical rationale for the selection of study topics. There is no plausible or widely accepted theory of sexual behaviour to act as a guide. Admittedly, there was no shortage of theoretical frameworks for the study of risk behaviour and behavioural change, derived mainly from social psychology. But most such models take an extremely rationalistic view of behaviour and their record in the prediction of behavioural outcomes is very mixed. It would have been folly to pin an expensive research endeavour, spanning many countries and half a decade, on any particular theory or model. As stated in Chapter 4, the overriding priority was to provide a description of behaviours, knowledge and beliefs that might be relevant to HIV transmission and thereby guide public information campaigns. Quite correctly, the surveys were designed more for an audience of programme managers than for academics.

How then have the WHO/GPA model questionnaires stood the test of time and analytic scrutiny? What improvements can be suggested? In addressing these questions, both the advantages and limitations of large scale cross-sectional surveys compared to smaller, more intensive studies should be kept firmly in mind. Surveys are potentially well suited to describing the climate of opinion and beliefs, to estimating the incidence of clearly specified behaviours, such as sexual intercourse outside marriage or use of condoms. Conversely, they are ill-suited to the elucidation of motivations that underlie behaviour, to the measurement of intensity of feelings, to the examination of behavioural change (a topic to which we shall return later), to the assessment of social interchanges or sexual networks or to provide satisfying explanations of behaviour. For adequate investigation of these and many other issues, complementary non-survey approaches are needed. WHO/GPA recognized from the outset that only a range of research methods could meet the needs for information and understanding arising from the HIV pandemic and had no hesitation in promoting other research studies that would complement standardized surveys.

The purpose of this discussion on the relative merits of different research methods is to emphasize that it is inappropriate to criticize the surveys for a failure to achieve results or insights for which they were never designed, or for which they were intrinsically inappropriate. It would be equally pointless to criticize small scale studies in single communities for lack of national representativeness.

The most important defect concerns a topic that is central to the stated objective of PR surveys, (though more peripheral to KABP enquiries) and lies well within the legitimate domain of the survey method. Expressed in blunt terms, PR surveys do not provide a fully adequate descriptive map of sexual partnerships. The approach has been described in Chapter 4 and hence only the bare outlines need to be repeated here. A primary distinction was made between regular partners (defined in terms of relative perman- ence) and others. Subsequently respondents were asked whether they had sexual contact with any non-regular partner in the last 12 months and, if so, how many. Further questions elicited whether the respondent had given money, gifts or favours in return for sex and, if so, whether this had occurred *always*, *sometimes* or *rarely* in the last 12 months.

Some elements of this definitional and measurement sequence are ap- propriate. It is surely correct to define and establish regular partnerships before proceeding to other sexual relationships. The use of a 12-month reference period cannot be faulted. But the sexual map or typology that emerges is infuriatingly imprecise. First, we learn next to nothing about the characteristics of regular partnerships, particularly when more than one is reported. It would not have been beyond the scope of a survey to collect key characteristics of each current regular partner in terms of duration, co- residence, childbearing, frequency of contact and so on. In so far as non- marital sex needs to be interpreted in the light of the nature of enduring partnerships, the approach falls a long way short of requirements.

A more critical defect is the failure to address properly the extremely complicated issue of sexual relationships that involve the transfer of money, gifts or favours. The variety of sexual exchanges that can occur is very wide and it is unrealistic to expect standardized surveys to capture the many subtle distinctions. Nevertheless, the failure to distinguish commercial sexual con- tacts from other relationships that might have some economic underpinning was an error of judgement. The former can be distinguished by an element of anonymity, payment of cash and by the respondent's belief that the sale of sexual favours forms an important source of income. Representative sur- veys of the adult population provide a good opportunity to collect informa- tion about commercial sex clients, though they are totally unsuited for investigation of sex workers themselves.

The importance of this distinction between contacts with sex workers and contacts with other non-regular partners is twofold. First, sex workers and their clients may be critical to the early spread of HIV. Second, such workers may be relatively easy to identify for focused interventions that will protect them, and their clients and thus diminish transmission. The failure of the surveys to provide the most accurate possible estimates of the inci- dence and circumstances (e.g., condom use) of commercial sex thus limits the utility of the findings for programme guidance.

Other methodological lessons have been mentioned in earlier chapters. The discussion in Chapter 2 reveals that some surveys used ambiguous euphemisms in translated versions of questionnaires that may have reduced cross-survey comparability of results. In Chapter 5, the point is made that access to condoms should be measured by objective or area reconnaissance as well as by questioning of individuals. The discussion in Chapter 6 makes it clear that the attempt to measure behavioural change was not a great success and that data on perceived personal risk or vulnerability are difficult to interpret.

In most other regards, however, WHO/GPA protocols have stood up well to scrutiny. The most obvious testimony is contained in this volume, which represents a huge advance in knowledge about sexual behaviour, condoms, and beliefs about AIDS in a diversity of settings.

Future Directions for AIDS-related Surveys of General Populations

As mentioned earlier, the HIV pandemic has created a wide range of research priorities that can only be met by a diversity of disciplines and research methods. It is inappropriate here to attempt to enumerate and discuss all main priorities. Instead the aim of this final section is a more modest and realistic one of identifying future directions for AIDS-related surveys of general populations.

The unique and crucial contribution that can be made by general population surveys depends on repetition of surveys that use comparable sampling frames and methods of measurement. If this strategy is followed, surveys will prove valuable in the monitoring of change, and thus act as a powerful tool for evaluating HIV-prevention programmes. As has been re-iterated several times in this volume, behavioural modification is the only way to check the spread of HIV pending the discovery of an effective vaccine or therapy. The required modifications include greater use of condoms and/or avoidance of unprotected intercourse with persons at risk of infection. Reduction of the incidence and prevalence of infection with other sexually transmitted diseases also merits mention as a further preventive strategy.

Repeated high quality surveys represent the only feasible way of finding out whether sexual behaviour among the general population is changing in desired directions. The main alternatives – prospective or cohort studies – provide more penetrating insights into behavioural change through periodic measures on the same individuals. But the cost and complexity of prospective studies with national coverage make this option unrealistic in most settings. Other alternatives, for instance the monitoring of condom sales or number of patients with sexually transmitted diseases, may prove valuable (and relatively cheap) but are no substitute for direct information on risk behaviours.

A useful analogy can be made at this juncture between family planning and HIV control programmes. Repeated cross-sectional surveys on family planning have proved indispensable in charting progress towards higher knowledge of methods, greater access and increased use of them. Without the objective evidence of progress that surveys provided, it is most unlikely that international funding for family planning would have been maintained at such a high level for so long. The history of family planning surveys, however, is a chequered one. In the 1960s, and early 1970s, study of the topic was dominated by knowledge, attitude and practice (KAP) surveys that varied in quality, coverage and content. Their results were greeted with considerable and justified scepticism (e.g., Hauser, 1967). Partly in response, the World Fertility Survey (WFS) programme was created in 1972 to conduct mutually comparable high quality surveys in developing countries. The WFS restored the credibility of the survey method and its successor, the Demographic and Health Survey (DHS) project, has continued the work. The substantive scope of surveys has widened so that the DHS now provides indicators of health and nutrition in addition to measures of contraception and demographic outcomes. The lesson for HIV programme evaluation is clear. Poorly designed, badly executed and underfunded surveys are useless, because the credibility of their results is too low for serious programme evaluation and resource allocation. Conversely, high quality surveys could be indispensable in demonstrating that the millions of dollars spent on HIV control are having some effect.

In both WFS and DHS projects, quality has implied a high price. The cost of a typical survey lies in the range of US$ 0.2 to 0.5 millions, and in developing countries there is heavy reliance on expensive foreign technical inputs. It is unlikely that HIV/AIDS evaluation can command resources of a similar magnitude. The correct response to this dilemma is to design HIV-evaluation surveys that are more simple in content and smaller in size than DHS-style surveys but not to make any sacrifices in terms of quality of design or execution. DHS samples are usually in the range of 5000 to 10,000 individuals, questionnaires usually occupy 30 to 50 pages and generate several hundred variables. Regularly repeated surveys on risk behaviours relevant to HIV and related knowledge and attitudinal items need cover no more than 30 or so key variables, with a questionnaire of a mere ten pages. The issue of sample size is more problematic, because decisions depend on the level of regional disaggregation required. Preliminary calculations suggest that a sample of 1000 men and 1000 women for each region, or domain, would be sufficiently large to detect, with 95 per cent confidence and power, a 10 per cent absolute increase in condom use or a similar decrease in the proportion reporting unprotected non-marital sex in the last 12 months. A total sample size of only 2000 would thus probably suffice if estimates of change at the national level only were required. A sample survey of this size and scope might cost between $50,000 and $100,000. If repeated every four years this seems a modest price in a country with a serious HIV/AIDS problem and where expenditures on HIV prevention may amount to hundreds of thousands of dollars per year.

In concentrating on the value of repeated surveys for monitoring and evaluation purposes, we do not intend to imply that they can serve no other valuable functions. On the contrary, the survey method, alone or in conjunction with smaller scale intensive enquiries, will continue to play a central role in further investigations of such key topics as risk perception, determinants of condom use, inter-partner communication and so on. Even in terms of straightforward descriptions of sexual partnerships, the WHO/GPA surveys mark only a start. As suggested earlier in this chapter, future surveys can and should do a much better job of specifying and measuring different types of sexual relationships, each of which may have different implications for risk taking and HIV transmission.

Thus far in the discussion, the issue of the reliability of survey data on sexual behaviour has been ignored. All that has been said in favour of surveys as tools of monitoring or evaluation or in other contexts is conditional upon their ability to yield data of reasonable reliability and validity. Objective, external validation of self-reported sexual behaviours is, in most contexts, impossible. But there are many other ways in which the quality of information can be assessed: internal consistency, inter-partner consistency, test-retest reliability, comparison of results of different data capture techniques and so on. There is a rapidly growing body of relevant evidence but nearly all methodological studies have been conducted in industrialized countries (Miller, *et al.*, 1990; Catania, *et al.*, 1990). In general, the results are encouraging; survey data on sexual behaviour are usually plausible, consistent, and reasonably reliable, though the differential reporting of numbers of sexual partners by men and women remains a serious and unresolved problem (e.g., Morris, 1993). However, it would be unjustified to assume that data of the same quality can be obtained in developing regions as have been obtained in Europe and North America.

Much remains to be learnt about the prevalence, the determinants and the social meanings of sexual behaviours. It is clear that surveys focusing on individual behaviour and their determinants, such as the 16 surveys presented in this volume, have their limits in HIV/AIDS prevention. They are inadequate in dealing with environmental and contextual factors such as political, social and economic determinants of risk-taking behaviour. Successful prevention strategies will require both changing individual behaviour and changing the social environment to support such behaviour change. A better understanding of individual and contextual factors, and of the interaction between the two, requires the development of methodological and paradigmatic triangulation of research approaches and methods, mixing qualitative and quantitative studies.

All techniques encounter problems of data quality; however prospective surveys on sexual behaviour are needed particularly to monitor change and evaluate programmes as well as search for new directions for interventions. The questionnaires have to be shorter, more focused on certain issues relevant to the local context, containing series of questions to better probe into certain topics which have not yet been fully understood. In the future KABP-type surveys are probably not so necessary; future studies need to be focused on sexual behaviour itself and on its social and economic determinants. In this way, AIDS programme managers can obtain clearer pictures of what is going on in their countries, and can draw the proper policy inferences to fight more efficiently HIV/AIDS.

Notes on Authors and Contributors

The multisite surveys described in this volume were coordinated first by the Social and Behavioural Research Unit (SBR) of the World Health Organization's Global Programme on AIDS (GPA), and subsequently by the Social and Behavioural Studies and Support Unit (SSB).

Michel Caraël is a member of the Surveillance, Evaluation and Forecasting Unit within the World Health Organization's Global Programme on AIDS. He was a member of the Social and Behavioural Research Unit between 1987 and 1990, and contributed to the development of the survey instruments used, and their implementation in the field.

Manuel Carballo was the head of the Social and Behavioural Research Unit within the World Health Organization's Global Programme on AIDS between 1987–1990.

John Cleland is Professor of Medical Demography at the London School of Hygiene and Tropical Medicine. He assisted in the design of the study instruments, and provided technical support to a number of studies in the field.

Jean-Claude Deheneffe of SONECOM, Belgium provided technical support for a number of studies in the field and in data management and processing.

Benoît Ferry is a member of the Social and Behavioural Studies and Support Unit of the World Health Organization's Global Programme on AIDS. He is on secondment to the Institut Français de Recherche Scientifique pour le Développement en Coopération (ORSTOM). He was responsible for monitoring the studies and coordinating data management and analysis.

Roger Ingham is Director of the Centre for Sexual Health Research at the University of Southampton, England. He has been a temporary adviser and consultant to the Social and Behavioural Studies and Support Unit of the World Health Organization's Global Programme on AIDS.

Masuma Mamdani is an epidemiologist who worked at the London School of Hygiene and Tropical Medicine from 1985 to 1993. She is now a freelance consultant in Baroda, India.

Amir Mehryar was a member of the Social and Behavioural Research Unit of the World Health Organization's Global Programme on AIDS between

1989–1991, and contributed to the development of the knowledge, attitude, belief and practice (KABP) instruments described in this volume. He is currently Deputy Director of the Institute for Research in Planning and Development, Tehran, Iran.

******

The tables and figures in the volume were produced by Jean-Claude Deheneffe and Jane Verrall, Short-Term Consultant to the Social and Behavioural Studies and Support Unit of the World Health Organization's Global Programme on AIDS. The regression analyses were undertaken by David Holmes, Lecturer in the Department of Statistics at the University of Southampton, England. The manuscript was prepared for publication by Julie Dew, Eva Rodrigues and Sylvie Schaller.

******

The in-country surveys described here were conducted in Brazil by Richard G. Parker of the Institute of Social Medicine at the State University of Rio de Janeiro; in Burundi by Nicéphore Ndimurukundo at the University of Burundi in Bujumbura; in the Central African Republic by Pierre Somsé, Head of the National Programme on AIDS; in Côte d'Ivoire by Seri Dedy, sociologist at the Institut d'Ethno-Sociologie of the Université d'Abidjan, and Gozé Tapé, psychologist at the Ecole Normale Supérieure, Abidjan; in Guinea Bissau by Juan Marcos of the CESTAS (Italy), who was project coordinator of an EEC funded technical support project to the National AIDS Programme in Guinea Bissau; in Kenya by Philista Onyango and P. Waliji-Moloo of the Department of Sociology at the University of Nairobi; in Lesotho by Agathe Lawson as a Short-Term Consultant for the World Health Organization's Global Programme on AIDS; in Mauritius by Clément Chan Kam, then National AIDS Programme manager; in the Philippines by Teodora V. Tiglao of the College of Public Health at the University of the Philippines; in Singapore by Kok Lee Peng of the Department of Psychological Medicine at the National University Hospital and by Ong Yong Wan, Chair of the AIDS Task Force of the Ministry of Health; in Sri Lanka by A.J. Weeramunda, senior lecturer in the Department of Sociology at the University of Colombo; in Tanzania by Eustace Muhondwa, now Director of the Institute of Public Health at Muhimbili University College of Health Sciences, M.T. Leshabari now head of the Behavioural Sciences Department in the Institute of Public Health at Muhimbili University College of Health Sciences, and by Y. Bwatwa, head of the department of Adult Education at the University of Dar-es-Salaam; in Thailand by Werasit Sittitrai of the Program on AIDS of the Thai Red Cross Society; in Togo by Geneviève Awissi, Chief of the Philosophy and Applied Social Sciences Department at the Université du Bénin; and in Zambia by Katele Kalumba of the Department of Community Medicine at the University of Zambia (currently Deputy Minister of Health) and by Alan Haworth of the Department of Psychiatry at the University of Zambia.

******

Review of this volume was undertaken by Peter Aggleton, Chief of the Social and Behavioural Studies and Support Unit within the Division of Research and Intervention Development of the World Health Organization's Global Programme on AIDS; Alix Adrien (Centre for AIDS Studies, Montréal General Hospital); Allan Hill (Center for Population and Development Studies, Harvard School of Public Health, Boston); Philippe Lehmann (AIDS Secretariat of the Office Fédéral de la Santé Publique, Berne); Thomas Coates (Center for AIDS Prevention Studies, University of California, San Francisco); Jean-Paul Moatti (Institut National de la Santé et de la Recherche Médicale (INSERM), Marseille) and Robert Tielman (University of Utrecht).

References

ACSF INVESTIGATORS (1992) 'AIDS and sexual behaviour in France', *Nature*, **360**, 407–9.

ADRIEN, A., CAYEMITTES, M., BERGEVIN, Y. (1993) 'AIDS-related knowledge, Attitudes, Beliefs and Practices in Haiti', *Bulletin of PAHO*, **27**, 3, 234–43.

AJZEN, I. and FISHBEIN, M. (1980) *Understanding Attitudes and Predicting Social Behaviour*, Englewood-Cliffs, NY: Prentice-Hall.

AJZEN, I. (1988) *Attitudes, Personality and Behaviour*, Milton Keynes: Open University Press.

ALLARD, R. (1989) Beliefs about AIDS as determinants of preventive practices and of support for coercive measures, *American Journal of Public Health*, **79**, 448–52.

AMERICAN PUBLIC HEALTH ASSOCIATION, FAMILY HEALTH INTERNATIONAL AND THE CENTERS FOR DISEASE CONTROL (1988) Condoms for prevention of sexually transmitted diseases, *Morbidity and Mortality Weekly Report*, **37**, 133–7.

ANDERSON, R.M. (1992) 'The transmission dynamics of sexually transmitted diseases: The behavioural component', in DYSON, T. (Ed.) *Sexual Behaviour and Networking: An Anthropological and Socio-cultural Studies on the Transmission of HIV*, Liege, Belgium: IUSSP, Derouaux Ordina Editions.

ANDERSON, R.M., MAY, R.M., BOILY, M.C., GARNETT, G.P. and ROWLEY, J.T. (1991) The spread of HIV-1 in Africa: sexual contact pattern and the predicted demographic impact of AIDS, *Nature*, **352**, 581–9.

BARONGO, L.R., BORGDORFF, M.W. *et al.* (1992) 'The epidemiology of HIV-1 infection in urban areas, roadside settlements and rural villages in Mwanza Region, Tanzania', *AIDS*, **6**, 1521–8.

BASNAYAKE, S. (1986) 'Knowledge and attitudes about reproductive health among youth in Sri Lanka', *Family Planning Association of Sri-Lanka*, **86**, 1.

BECKER, M.H. (Ed.) (1974) 'The health belief model and personal health behaviour', *Health Education Monographs*, **2**, 324–508.

BLANC, A.K. and RUTENBERG, N. (1990) 'Assessment of the quality of data on age at first sexual intercourse, age at first marriage and age at first birth in demographic and health surveys', *Demographic and Health Surveys Methodological Reports*, No. 1. Columbia, MD: Institute for Resource Development.

BLANC, A.K. and RUTENBERG, N. (1991) 'Coitus and contraception: The utility of data on sexual intercourse for family planning programs', *Studies in Family Planning*, **22**, 3, 162–76.

BLENDON, R.J. and DONELAN, K. (1988) 'Discrimination against people with AIDS: The public's perspectives', *New England Journal of Medicine*, **319**, 1022–6.

BRORRSON, B. and HERLITZ, C. (1988) 'The AIDS epidemic in Sweden: Changes in awareness, attitudes and behaviour', *Scandinavian Journal of Social Medicine*, **16**, 67–71.

BROWN, L.K., DI CLEMENTE, R.J. and REYNOLDS, L.A. (1991) 'HIV prevention for adolescents: Utility of the health belief model', *AIDS Education and Prevention*, **3**, 1, 50–9.

CALDWELL, J.C. and CALDWELL, P. (1986) 'Is the Asian family planning program model suited to Africa?', *Studies in Family Planning*, **19**, 1, 19–28.

CALDWELL, J.C., CALDWELL, P. and QUIGGIN, P. (1989) 'The social context of AIDS in Sub-Saharan Africa', *Population and Development Review*, **15**, 2, 185–234.

CALDWELL, J.C., ORUBULOYE, I.O. and CALDWELL, P. (1992) 'Underreaction to AIDS in Sub-Saharan Africa', *Social Science and Medicine*, **34**, 1169–82.

CAPRON, J. and KOHLER, J. (1975) Migration de travail et pratique matrimoniale. Migration à partir du pays Mossi, Mimeo, Ouagadougou, Burkina Faso, ORSTOM.

CARAËL, M. (1987) 'Le Sida en Afrique', in HIRSCH, E. (Ed.) *Le Sida, Rumeurs et Faits*. Paris: Les Editions du Cerf. 53–66.

CARAËL, M. (1993) 'Women's vulnerability to STD/HIV in Sub-Saharan Africa: Increasing evidence', Paper presented at a seminar on Women and Demographic Change in Sub-Saharan Africa, IUSSP, Dakar, 3–6 March.

CARAËL, M. (1994) 'The impact of change in marriage on STD and HIV', in BLEDSOE, C. and PISON, G. (Eds) *Nuptiality in Sub-Saharan Africa: Current Changes and Impact on Fertility*, Oxford: Oxford University Press.

CATANIA, J., GIBSON, D., CHITWOOD, D. and COATES, T. (1990) 'Methodological problems in AIDS behavioral research: Influence on measurement error and participation bias in studies of sexual behavior', *Psychological Bulletin*, **108**, 3, 339–62.

CLELAND, J. and VAN GINNEKEN, J. (1989) 'Maternal schooling and childhood mortality', *Journal of the Biosocial Sciences*, Suppl. 10, 13–34.

CONANT, M., HARDY, D., SERNATINGER, J., SPICER, D. and LEVY, J.A. (1986) 'Condoms prevent transmission of AIDS-associated Retrovirus', *Journal of the American Medical Association*, **255**, 1706.

COXON, A. (1988) 'The number game: Gay lifestyles, epidemiology of AIDS and social science', in AGGLETON, P. and HOMANS, H. (Eds) *Social Aspects of AIDS*, Lewes, Falmer Press.

DAB, W., MOATTI, J.P., BASTIDE, S., ABENHAÏM, L. and BRUNET, J.B. (1989) 'Misconceptions about transmission of AIDS and attitudes toward prevention in French general public', *AIDS*, **3**, 433–7.

DARE, L.O. and CLELAND, J. (1993) 'Reliability and validity of survey data on sexual behaviour: Preliminary results of field test', Paper presented at the IUSSP seminar on AIDS Impact and Prevention in the Developing World: the contribution of demography and social science, Annecy (France).

DIRECTION DE LA STATISTIQUE (1984) 'Enquête Nationale Ivoirienne sur la Fécondité 1980–81, Rapport Principal', Abidjan, Direction de la Statistique.

DIXON-MUELLER, R. and WASSERHEIT, J. (1990) 'The culture of silence: Reproductive tract infections among women in the third world', New York: International Women's Health Coalition.

FATHALLAH, M.F. (1990) Relationship between contraceptive technology and HIV transmission: An overview. In ALEXANDER, N.J., GABELNICK, H.L. and SPIELER, J.M. (Eds) *Heterosexual Transmission of AIDS*, New York: Wiley-Liss, 225–34.

FAULKENBERRY, J.R., VINCENT, M., JAMES, A. and JOHNSON, W. (1987) 'Coital behaviours, attitudes and knowledge of students who experience early coitus', *Adolescence*, **22**, 321–32.

FELDBLUM, P.J. and FORTNEY, J.A. (1988) 'Condoms, spermicides and the transmission of human immunodeficiency virus: A review of the literature', *American Journal of Public Health*, **78**, 52–4.

FEYISITAN, B. and PEBLEY, A.R. (1989) 'Pre-marital sexuality in urban Nigeria', *Studies in Family Planning*, **20**, 6, 343–54.

FINCH, B.E. and GREEN, H. (1963) *Contraception Through the Ages*. Springfield, IL: Charles C. Thomas.

FISHBEIN, M. and AJZEN, I. (1975) *Belief, Attitude, Intention and Behaviour: An Introduction to Theory and Research*. Reading, MA: Addison-Wesley.

FRANK, O. (1987) 'The demand for fertility control in sub-Saharan Africa', *Studies in Family Planning*, **18**, 4, 181–201.

GOLDBERG, H.I., LEE, N.C., OBERLE, M.W. and PETERSON, H.B. (1989) 'Knowledge about condoms and their use in less developed countries during a period of rising AIDS prevalence', *Bulletin of the World Health Organization*, **67**, 1, 85–91.

HARDY, A.M. (1990) 'National health interview survey data on adult knowledge of AIDS in the United States', *Public Health Reports*, **6**, 629–34.

HAUSER, P. (1967) 'Family planning and population programs', (Review). *Demography*, **4**.

HINGSON, R.W., STRUNIN, L., BERLIN, B.M. and HEEREN, T. (1990) 'Beliefs about AIDS, use of alcohol and drugs and unprotected sex amongst Massachusetts adolescents', *American Journal of Public Health*, **80**, 295–9.

HOGAN, T. (1989) 'Psychophysical relation between perceived threat of AIDS and willingness to impose social restrictions', *Health Psychology*, **8**, 255–66.

INGHAM, R. (1994) 'Some speculations on the concept of rationality', in ALBRECHT, G. (Ed.) *Advances in Medical Sociology*, **4**, Greenwich, CT: JAI Press.

INGHAM, R. and HOLMES, D. (1991) 'Comparative analysis of KABP surveys conducted in four countries: Kenya, Singapore, Mauritius, Central African Republic', Southampton, UK. Geneva, Social and Behavioural Studies and Support Unit, Global Programme on AIDS, World Health Organization, 176 p. (Draft).

INGHAM, R. and VAN ZESSEN, G. (1994) 'Towards an alternative model of sexual behaviour: From individual properties to interactional processes', Unpublished paper to appear as chapter in a book to be prepared by an EC Concerted Action on Sexual Behaviour, (coordinated by M. Hubert, Brussels).

JOHNSON, A.M., WADSWORTH, J., WELLINGS, K., BRADSHAW, S. and FIELD, J. (1992) 'Sexual lifestyles and HIV risk', *Nature*, **360**, 410–12.

KAMENGA, M., JINGU, K. and HASSIG, S., NDILU, M., BEHETS, F., BROWN, C. and RYDER, R. (1989) 'Condom use and associated HIV-sero-conversion following intensive HIV counselling of 122 married couples in Zaire with discordant HIV serology', Paper presented at the Vth International Conference on AIDS, Montreal, June 1989 (Abstract TDO35).

KINSEY, A.C., POMEROY, W. and MARTIN, C. (1948) *Sexual Behaviour in Human Male*, Philadelphia, PA: Sanders.

KINSEY, A.C., POMEROY, W. and MARTIN, C. (1953) *Sexual Behaviour in Human Female*. Philadelphia, PA: Sanders.

KNOLLE, H. (1991) 'A model to assess the impact of traditional sexual standards on the spread of AIDS in Africa.' Poster MD 4100. Presentation at the VIIth International Conference on AIDS, Florence.

KONINGS, E., ANDERSON, R.M., LEVIN, A., SISO, Z., BRUBAKER, G. and BLATTNER, W. (1994) 'Patterns of Heterosexual Behaviour in a Rural Community in North West Tanzania', Submitted for publication.

LANDE, R. (1993) 'Controlling sexually transmitted diseases', *Population Reports*. Series L. No. 9.

LARSON, A. (1989) 'Social context of HIV transmission in Africa: Historical and cultural bases of east and central African sexual relations', *Review of Infectious Diseases*, **2**, 5, 716–31.

LESTHAEGHE, R.J. (Ed.) (1989) *Reproduction and Social Organization in Sub-Saharan Africa.* Berkeley, CA: University of California Press.

LÉVI-STRAUSS, C. (1949) *Les Structures Élémentaires de la Parenté.* Paris, Presses Universitaires de France.

LINDAN, C., ALLEN, S., CARAËL, M., NSENGUMUREMYI, F., VAN DE PERRE, P., SERUFILIRA, A., TICE, J., BLACK, D., COATES, T. and HULLEY, S. (1991) 'Knowledge, attitudes and perceived risk of AIDS among urban Rwandan women: Relationships to HIV infection and behaviour change', *AIDS*, **5**, 993–1002.

LISKIN, L. *et al.* (1990) 'Condoms – now more than ever', *Population Reports*. Series H, No. 8.

LITTLE, K. (1973) *African Women in Towns: An Aspect of Africa's Social Revolution,* London: Cambridge University Press.

LOEWENSTEIN, G. and FURSTENBERG, F. (1991) 'Is teenage sexual behaviour rational?', *Journal of Applied Social Psychology*, **21**, 957–86.

LONDON, K.A., CUSHING, J., RUSTEIN, S.O., CLELAND, D.J., ANDERSON, J.E., MORIRIS, L. and MOORE, S.H. (1985) 'Fertility and family planning surveys: An update', *Population Reports*, Series M, No. 8.

MAIMAN, L.A. and BECKER, M.H. (1974) 'The health belief model: Origins and correlates in psychological theory'. In BECKER, M.H. (Ed.) *The Health Belief Model and Personal Health Behaviour.* Thorofare, NJ: Charles B. Slack, Inc.

MALINOWSKI, B. (1929) *The Sexual Life of Savages,* New York: Harcourt Brace Jovanovich.

MAMDANI, M., CLELAND, J. and IBO, M.M. (1991) 'Assessment of quality of WHO survey data on sexual behaviour in Central African Republic, Kenya, Ivory Coast, Mauritius, Singapore and Togo', London School of Hygiene and Tropical Medicine, Unpublished paper.

MANN, J., QUINN, T.C. and PIOT, P. *et al.* (1986) 'Condom use and HIV infection among prostitutes in Zaire', *New England Journal of Medicine*, **316**, 345.

MEAD, M. (1949) *Male and Female: A Study of Sexes in a Changing World.* New York: W. Morrow.

MEILLASSOUX, C. (1975) *Femmes, Greniers et Capitaux.* Paris: Maspéro.

MERTENS, T., CARAËL, M., SATO, P., CLELAND, J., WARD, H. and SMITH, G.D. (1994) 'Evaluation progress towards implementation of the global AIDS strategy', *AIDS*, **8**, 361–72.

MILLER, H.G., TURNER, C.F. and MOSES, L.E. (Eds) (1990) *Methodological Issues in AIDS Surveys.* Washington, DC: National Academy Press.

MOATTI, J.P., DAB, W., LOUNDOU, A., QUENEL, P., BELTZER, N., ANES, A. and POLLAK, M. (1992) 'Impact of media campaigns against AIDS in the general public: A French evaluation', *Health Policy*, **21**, 233–47.

MOATTI, J.P., DAB, W., POLLAK, M. (1992) 'Les Français et le Sida . . . les comportements changent', *La Recherche*. **23**, 247, 1202–11.

MONTGOMERY, S.B., JOSEPH, J.G., BECKER, M.H., OSTROW, D.G., KESSLER, R.C. and KIRSCHT, J.P. (1989) 'The health belief model in understanding compliance with preventative recommendations for AIDS: How useful?', *AIDS Education and Prevention*, **1**, 303–23.

MORRIS, L. (1990) 'Sexual experience and use of contraception among young adults in Latin America', Presented at the Annual Meeting of the Population Association of America, Toronto.

MORRIS, M. (1993) 'Telling Tails Explain the Discrepancy in Sexual Partner Reports', *Nature*, **365**, 437–40.

MOSHA, F., NICOLL, A., BARONGO, L., BORGDORFF, M., NEWELL, J., SENKORO, K., GROSSKURTH, H., CHANGALUCHA, J., KLOKKE, A. and KILLEWO, J. (1993) 'A population-based study of syphilis and sexually transmitted disease syndromes in Northwestern Tanzania. 1-Prevalence and incidence', *Genitourinary Medicine*, **69**, 415–20.

MURRAY, C. (1977) 'High bridewealth, migrant labour and the position of women in Lesotho', *Journal of African Law*, **21**, 1, 79–96.

NGUGI, E.N., PLUMMER, F.A., SIMONSEN, J.N., CAMERON, D.W., BOSIRE, M., WAIYAKI, P., RONALD, A.R. and NDINYA-ACHOLA, J.O. (1988) 'Prevention of transmission of human immunodeficiency virus in Africa: Effectiveness of condom promotion and health education among prostitutes', *Lancet*, ii, 887–90.

PARKIN, D. and NYAMWAYA, D. (Eds) (1987) *Transformations of African Marriage*. Manchester: Manchester University Press for the International African Institute.

PAUL, J., CROSBY, G.M., MIDANIK, L. and STALL, R. (1991) 'A new method of measuring the association between alcohol/drug use and high risk sex', Paper presented at the VIIth International Conference on AIDS, Florence, Italy, (abstract MD 4044).

PNLS (1991) Enquête nationale de séroprévalence au VIH. Programme national de lutte contre le Sida. Ministère de la Santé. Bujumbura, document dactylographié.

POLLAK, M. and MOATTI, J.P. (1989) 'HIV-Risk Perception and Determinants of Sexual Behaviour', in HUBERT, M. (Ed.) *Sexual Behaviour and Risks of HIV Infection*, Bruxelles, Facultés Universitaires Saint-Louis.

RADCLIFFE-BROWN, A.R. and FORDE, D. (Eds) (1987) *African Systems of Kinship and Marriage*, London: Oxford University Press for the International African Institute.

RIETMEIJER, C.A.M., KROBER, J.W., FCORNIO, P.M. and JUDSON, F.N. (1988) 'Condoms as physical and chemical barriers against human immunodeficiency virus', *Journal of the American Medical Association*, **259**, 1851–3.

RISE, J., KRAFT, P. and JAKOBSEN, R. (1991) 'HIV-related attitudes and knowledge of HIV transmission in Norway', Paper presented at First Conference on Biopsychosocial Aspects of HIV Infection, Amsterdam, 22–25 September.

ROSENSTOCK, I.M. (1974) 'Historical origins of the health belief model', *Health Education Monographs*, **2**, 328–35.

ROSENSTOCK, I.M., STRECHER, V.J. and BECKER, M.H. (1988) 'Social learning theory and the health belief model', *Health Education Quarterly*, **15**, 175–83.

ROSS, T.A., RICH, M., MOLZAN, J.P. and PENSAK, M. (1988) *Family planning and child survival: 100 Developing Countries*, New York: Columbia University Center for Population and Family Health.

ROTTER, J.B. (1966) 'Generalized expectancies for internal versus external control of reinforcement', *Psychological Monographs*, **80**, 609.

SARWONO, S.W. (1983) *The Problem of Adolescent Fertility in Indonesia*, London, IPPF.

SCHULZ, K.F., CATES, W. and O'MARA, P.R. (1987) 'Pregancy loss, infant death and suffering: Legacy of syphilis and gonorrhoea in Africa', *Genitourinary Medicine*, **63**, 5, 320–5.

SHERRIS, J.D. *et al.* (1982) 'Update on condoms – products, protection, promotion'. *Population Reports*, Series H, No. 6.

SITTITRAI, W. and BARRY, J. (1990) 'Research on human sexuality in pattern III countries', in CHOUINARD, A. and ALBERT, J. (Eds) *Human Sexuality: Research Perspectives in a World Facing AIDS*, Ottawa: IRDC, 173–90.

SOKAL, D., LANKOANDE, S., MUGADITCHIAN, D., LAMIZANA, P., TREBUCQ, A., SALLA, R. and KAPTUE, L. (1992) The Use of Male STD History as an Indicator for Impact Assessment. In PACCAUD, F., J.P. VADER and GUTZWILLER, F. *Assessing AIDS Prevention*, Basel, Birkhäuser Verlag.

SPIRA, A., BAJOS, N. and GROUPE ACSF (1993) *Les comportements sexuels en France*, Paris: La Documentation Française.

STOLLER, E.J. and RUTHERFORD, W. (1989) Evaluation of AIDS Prevention and Control Programs, *AIDS*, **3**, S289-S296.

STANDING, H. and KISSEKA, M.N. (1989) Sexual Behaviour in Sub-Saharan Africa. An Annotated Bibliography, London: Report to the ODA.

TANQUARY, A.C. and WITTE, J.H. (1990) Condoms: Overview of Technology, Materials and Development. In ALEXANDER, N.J., GABELNICK, H.L. and SPIELER, J.M. (Eds) *Heterosexual Transmission of AIDS*, New York: Wiley-Liss.

UNITED NATIONS (1987) Fertility Behaviour in the Context of Development: Evidence from the World Fertility Survey, *Population Studies*, **100**.

UNITED NATIONS (1989) Adolescent Reproductive Behaviour (Volume II) *Population Studies*, **109**, Add.1.

UNITED NATIONS (1990a) *Demographic Year Book*, New York: Population Division.

UNITED NATIONS (1990b) *World Population Prospects* 1990, New York: Population Division.

UN/WHO (1991) The AIDS Epidemic and its Demographic Consequences, New York/Geneva: United Nations/World Health Organization.

URD-DHS (1989) Enquête Démographique et de Santé au Togo 1988, Lomé and Columbia (Unpublished).

VANCE, C.S. (1991) 'Anthropology rediscovers sexuality: A theoretical comment', *Social Science and Medicine*, **33**, 8, 875–884.

VAN DE PERRE, P., JACOBS, D. and SPRECHER-GOLDBERGER, S. (1987) 'The latex condom, an efficient barrier against sexual transmission of AIDS-related viruses', *AIDS*, **1**, 49–52.

WADSWORTH, J., FIELD, J., JOHNSON, A.M., BRADSHAW, S. and WELLINGS, K. (1993) 'Methodology of the national survey on sexual attitudes and lifestyles', *Journal of the Royal Statistical Society Series A: Statistics in Society*, **156**, 3, 407–21.

WA KARANJA, W. (1987) Outside Wives and Inside Wives in Nigeria: a study of changing perceptions in marriage. In PARKIN, D. and NYAMWAYA, D. (Eds) *Transformations of African Marriage*. Manchester, Manchester University Press.

WASSERHEIT, J.N. (1992) Epidemiological Synergy: interrelationships between human immunodeficiency virus infection and other sexually transmitted diseases. *Sexually Transmitted Diseases*, **19**, 2, 61–77.

WESTOFF, C.F. (1974) Coital Frequency and Contraception. *Family Planning Perspectives*, **6**, 3, 136–41.

WHO/GPA (1990a) *Knowledge, Attitudes, Beliefs and Practices on AIDS (KABP) Phase 1*: research package. Geneva, Social and Behavioural Research Unit, Global Programme on AIDS, World Health Organization. (Draft).

WHO/GPA (1990b) *Knowledge, Attitudes, Beliefs and Practices on AIDS (KABP) Phase 2*: research package. Geneva, Social and Behavioural Research Unit, Global Programme on AIDS, World Health Organization. (Draft).

WHO/GPA (1990c) *Partner Relations and Risk of HIV Infection (Phase 1)*: research package. Geneva, Social and Behavioural Research Unit, Global Programme on AIDS, World Health Organization. (Draft).

WHO/GPA (1990d) *Partner Relations and Risk of HIV Infection (Phase 2)*: research package. Geneva, Social and Behavioural Research Unit, Global Programme on AIDS, World Health Organization. (Draft).

WHO/GPA (1990e) *Combined Partner Relations/KABP Survey (Phase 2)*: research package. Geneva, Social and Behavioural Research Unit, Global Programme on AIDS, World Health Organization. (Draft).

WHO/GPA (1991) *Data Management Manual: KABP (Phase I)*. Geneva, Social and Behavioural Research Unit, Global Programme on AIDS, World Health Organization. (Draft).

WILKINS, H.A., ALONSO, P., BALDEH, S., CHAM, M.K., CORRAH, T., HUGHES, A., JAITEH, K.O., OELMAN, B. and PICKERING, H. (1989) 'Knowledge of AIDS, use of condoms and results of counselling subjects with asymptomatic HIV-2 infection in The Gambia', *AIDS Care*, 1, 3, 247–56.

WILSON, D., LAVELLE, S., MACHOKOTO, S. and ARMSTRONG, M. (1992) 'Use of a retrospective timeline calendar to examine alcohol use, sexual behaviour and condom use among Zimbabwean men' (Unpublished report), Harare: University of Zimbabwe.

WINKELSTEIN, W., LYMAN, D.M., PADIAN, N., GRANT, R., SAMUEL, M., WILEY, J.A., ANDERSON, R.E., LANG, W., RIGGS, J. and LEVY, J.A. (1987) 'Sexual practices and risk of HIV infection: The San Francisco men's health study', *Journal of the American Medical Association*, 257, 321–5.